Proton Therapy - Scientific Questions and Future Direction

Edited by Thomas J. FitzGerald

Published in London, United Kingdom

Proton Therapy - Scientific Questions and Future Direction
http://dx.doi.org/10.5772/intechopen.111250
Edited by Thomas J. FitzGerald

Contributors
Abdel Karim Ferouani, Abdessamad Sekkal, Alexander Levichev, Andrey Palyanov, Eter Natelauri, Linda Ding, Mariam Pkhaladze, Maryann Bishop-Jodoin, Mikhail Neshchadim, Mikheil Atskvereli, Mohammed Sahlaoui, Rafik Hazem, Thomas J. FitzGerald, Yulia Klevtsova

Notice

Statements and opinions expressed in the chapters are these of the individual contributors and not necessarily those of the editors or publisher. No responsibility is accepted for the accuracy of information contained in the published chapters. The publisher assumes no responsibility for any damage or injury to persons or property arising out of the use of any materials, instructions, methods or ideas contained in the book.

First published in London, United Kingdom, 2024 by IntechOpen
IntechOpen is the global imprint of INTECHOPEN LIMITED, registered in England and Wales, registration number: 11086078, 5 Princes Gate Court, London, SW7 2QJ, United Kingdom

British Library Cataloguing-in-Publication Data
A catalogue record for this book is available from the British Library

Additional hard and PDF copies can be obtained from orders@intechopen.com

Proton Therapy - Scientific Questions and Future Direction
Edited by Thomas J. FitzGerald
p. cm.
Print ISBN 978-0-85466-341-5
Online ISBN 978-0-85466-340-8
eBook (PDF) ISBN 978-0-85466-342-2

We are IntechOpen,
the world's leading publisher of
Open Access books
Built by scientists, for scientists

7,000+
Open access books available

186,000+
International authors and editors

200M+
Downloads

Our authors are among the

156
Countries delivered to

Top 1%
most cited scientists

12.2%
Contributors from top 500 universities

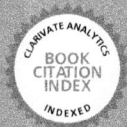

CLARIVATE ANALYTICS

BOOK
CITATION
INDEX

INDEXED

WEB OF SCIENCE™

Selection of our books indexed in the Book Citation Index
in Web of Science™ Core Collection (BKCI)

Interested in publishing with us?
Contact book.department@intechopen.com

Numbers displayed above are based on latest data collected.
For more information visit www.intechopen.com

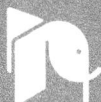

Meet the editor

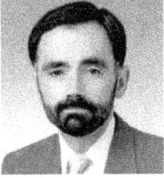

Dr. Thomas J. FitzGerald is a professor and chair of the University of Massachusetts Chan Medical School Department of Radiation Oncology and the director of the National Cancer Institute Imaging and Radiation Oncology Core (IROC) office in Lincoln, RI. In this capacity, Dr. FitzGerald serves as the quality assurance director for multiple cooperative groups within the National Clinical Trials Network (NCTN). Protons have become incorporated into NCTN clinical trials, especially in the pediatric domain, and IROC writes all clinical trials within the NCTN for proton care and reviews all patient data in real-time to ensure targets treated with both protons and photons meet compliance standards established for each trial.

Contents

Preface

Proton therapy for cancer patients is increasingly being used worldwide and becoming available in multiple centers. The miniaturization of proton technology has created an opportunity for many institutions to initiate plans for proton care. The ability to place a unit in the size of a therapy vault will further improve cost and permit the expansion of proton care to an enterprise level. As technology continues to improve, new questions arise about how to further improve technology and make centers more available. In this book, we evaluate outstanding scientific questions concerning proton care delivery and off insights into future directions for proton care. We appreciate your time and interest.

Thomas J. FitzGerald, MD
Department of Radiation Oncology,
UMass Chan Medical School,
Worcester, Massachusetts, USA

Chapter 1

Introductory Chapter: Proton Therapy – The Promise is Moving to an Enterprise Function

Linda Ding, Maryann Bishop-Jodoin and Thomas J. FitzGerald

1. Introduction

Radiation therapy has become increasingly important in the care of patients with cancer. Progress in radiation therapy technology has provided more opportunities to treat patients with curative intent. In multiple disease sites, patients with oligometastatic disease are treated with comprehensive radiation therapy to all sites of disease at presentation with improved outcomes. Common sense would argue that as additional sites of disease are treated in an increasingly comprehensive manner, more normal tissue would be unintentionally treated as part of the radiation therapy care plan which in turn could augment sequelae of management and limit the application of additional therapies. Mitigating this issue with improved radiation therapy treatment technology would serve to improve outcomes by assuring full dose to tumor target and decreased dose to normal tissue. Compared to photon-directed radiation treatment, proton-directed therapy can provide uniform radiation dose to tumor targets with decreased dose to normal tissue, thus improving the therapeutic index for patient care. The goal of radiation therapy is to provide tumor control with limited risk of injury and proton therapy serves as an ideal platform to ensure optimal outcomes. Based on the fundamental understanding that ionizing radiation transfers energy into tissues resulting in DNA damage leading to tissue injury and cell death, identifying pathways to limit normal tissue injury, and enhance tumor cell kill with systemic therapies improves patient outcomes. Because of the inherent capability of proton therapy limiting dose to normal tissue, defining pathways to facilitate the deployment of proton therapy worldwide will serve to improve patient outcomes moving forward. This has to be balanced with the cost of production and availability of expertise with the appropriate training to both initiate and maintain a proton program [1–6].

2. History

As is well demonstrated by atomic theory, atoms are comprised of particles with a positive charge (protons), a negative charge (electrons), and a neutral charge (neutrons). Robert Wilson was the first to recognize the medical application of proton therapy. Wilson recognized that protons exhibit a progressive change in velocity as they migrate through tissue and culminate in what is termed a "Bragg peak" with a rapid drop off in energy after the peak. The working premise was that by harnessing

IntechOpen

the geometry of the pathway and Bragg peak, protons could be used to target disease housed within and in close approximation to normal tissue. Because of the decrease in energy beyond the peak, normal tissue beyond the peak would only receive a nominal dose, unlike treatment plans using photons. His vision was prescient and far ahead of its time and remains a fundamental principle in patient care today with particle therapy.

Radiation therapy has a rich scientific history. William Roentgen developed a cathode ray tube which led to the discovery of X-rays. One of his many primary findings was that an X-ray can pass through solid objects however the fact the X-ray is significantly titrated by bone and metal remains a fundamental principle of radiology practice to this day. Becquerel discovered radioactivity and Marie Curie discovered radium which would build the bridge to medical sciences. From their seminal work, both diagnostic and therapy programs matured into now what is an extraordinary industry producing devices that generate high-energy beams re-purposed in a nimble and efficient manner for direct patient care. Expertise in medical care and medical physics has provided a pathway for unprecedented process improvements in patient outcomes with treatments today that are highly sophisticated, modulated by dynamic multi-leaf function during therapy, and aligned with targets with efficient and modern daily image guidance. The technology improvements within the past two decades are extraordinary with modern trainees unfamiliar with the processes and limitations of treating patients in the past. Applying the technology success in photon care to proton care is becoming an important next step for proton manufacturers and will lead to moving proton care into a worldwide enterprise function providing cost can be controlled and continued miniaturization of proton units can be designed and retrofitted into existing therapy vaults for cost savings [1–3, 6].

3. Future directions

To make proton care more available to the general population of oncology patients, continuous process improvements are required to both facilitate patient care and make proton care available to the global oncology community. Initial proton treatment facilities had multiple therapy gantries associated with the cyclotron/synchrotron and required large building footprints for treatment execution. Today, treatment facilities are being designed with less cost in a building footprint similar to a photon accelerator. This has led to significant changes in how proton centers are both designed and distributed worldwide. Single gantry systems developed by multiple vendors have significantly reduced the cost of developing a proton center. Currently, there are approximately 100 proton centers operational worldwide with more than 30 centers in Europe. The Roberts Proton Center at the University of Pennsylvania is one of the largest centers in the world housing multiple gantries for patient care. Washington University of St. Louis houses a single gantry system with a cost significantly less than a larger center making proton therapy accessible to many institutions and patients worldwide. Washington University has recently installed a second single gantry system due to the need to provide service to the larger community. The continued miniaturization of proton technology will continue to make the product less expensive bringing the technology within reach for institutions less capable of purchasing other larger systems. Vendors evaluating the possibility of placing a unit in an existing photon therapy vault. This effort includes clever design of the unit and novel table designs to treat patients in multiple positions with a table which can support patients in multiple sitting positions. These efforts represent significant advances in engineering making particle therapy available to an increasing number of institutions worldwide and accordingly, making proton therapy available to more patients. The transition to smaller, more affordable, units will provide a pathway to global applications of proton therapy. Proton manufacturers are working to bring all of the important elements of modern photon care into proton therapy treatment execution including image guidance and multi-leaf-based intensity modulation treatment execution. Aligning and coupling proton care treatment strategies with processes well known to photon physics teams and radiation therapists facilitates the transition of treatment staff to care for patients being treated with proton plans. As engineering is perfected, costs will decrease as the deployment of proton units moves to an enterprise level of distribution [6].

The types of patients and disease sites treated with proton therapy are rapidly increasing at an enterprise level. With the larger, more cumbersome early proton tools, beam compensation processes had to be applied on a daily basis for patient care and this served to limit the patient population treated and managed with proton care. Initially lesions in the central nervous system, then less amenable to surgical intervention including pituitary disease, were treated with protons. As facilities have increased in number and the patient care process in proton therapy delivery have become nimble, nearly every disease site in the treatment of the modern oncology patient has benefits when treated with protons as dose to normal tissue can be titrated in all body sites. Protons are no longer an eclectic therapy used in limited and selected disease sites. In adult oncology central nervous system, head/neck, thorax, upper/lower abdomen, pelvis, and extremity patients are now treated with proton therapy. Protocols are currently active comparing proton and photon care in multiple disease sites with tumor control and normal tissue endpoints designed to determine which sites benefit most from proton care. There is significant interest in expanding the use of proton applications in pediatric oncology patients. With 25% of pediatric oncology population of patients afflicted with disease in the central nervous system, proton applications are highly attractive. With modern imaging tools, the disease can be targeted with increasing accuracy further supporting the application of proton therapy with normal tissue conformal avoidance. Thoracic, abdominal, pelvic, and extremity disease sites in the pediatric population can be targeted with improved normal tissue conformal avoidance. In selected protocols in the Children's Oncology Group (COG), a significant percentage of patients treated with radiation therapy are treated with protons reflecting increased utilization of proton therapy worldwide [4–6].

Patients can be successfully treated with radiation therapy with photons or protons. Because of the improved dose distribution of protons to normal tissue, protons present a theoretical advantage to photons with respect to radiation dose to normal tissue. This can have an important consequence for patient management moving forward as radiation dose to normal tissue has an impact on supplemental care including targeted and systemic management. Continued process improvements including progress in miniaturization will further support the application of protons into daily patient care management.

In this chapter, we present theoretical and practical aspects of proton care management which have importance moving forward for proton application in patient care. Hopefully, with these and other changes, proton can move worldwide into enterprise function.

Author details

Linda Ding, Maryann Bishop-Jodoin and Thomas J. FitzGerald*
University of Massachusetts Chan Medical School, Worcester, MA, United States

*Address all correspondence to: tj.fitzgerald@umassmemorial.org

IntechOpen

References

[1] Suit H, Kooy H, Trofinov A, Farr J, Munzenrider J, DeLaney T, et al. Should positive phase 3 clinical trial data be required before proton beam therapy is more widely adopted? No. Radiotherapy and Oncology. 2008;**86**(2):148-153. DOI: 10.1016/j.rad.onc.2007.12.024

[2] Jagsi R, DeLaney T, Donelan K, Tarbell N. Real-time rationing of scarce resources: The Northeast Proton Therapy Experience. Journal of Clinical Oncology. 2004;**22**(11):2246-2250. DOI: 10.1200/JCO.2004.10.083

[3] Furlow B. Dosimetric promise versus cost: Critics question proton therapy. Lancet Oncology. 2013;**14**(9):805-806. DOI: 10.1016/s1470-2045(13)70314-0

[4] National Cancer Institute. Childhood Cancer Data Initiative 2020. Available from: https://www.cancer.gov/research/areas/childhood/childhood-cancer-data-initiative

[5] Bishr M, Zaghloul M. Radiation therapy availability in Africa and Latin America: Two models of low and middle income countries. International Journal of Radiation Oncology • Biology • Physics. 2018;**102**(3):490-498. DOI: 10.1016/j.ijrobp.2018.06.046

[6] Calvo MF, Panizo E, Matin S, Serrano J, Cambeiro M, Azcoma D, et al. Proton Cancer Therapy: Synchrotron-based Clinical Experiences 2020 in Proton Therapy-current Status and Future Directions. Vol. 2021. London, UK: IntechOpen; 2021. pp. 81-120. DOI: 10.5772/intechopen 91072

Chapter 2

Perspective Chapter: The Proton's Theoretical Description, Based on Wigner-Segal Approach to Elementary Particles

Yulia Klevtsova, Alexander Levichev, Mikhail Neshchadim and Andrey Palyanov

Abstract

The chapter focuses on the Multi-Level Model (MLM), a conceptual framework proposed by Levichev. The essence of the MLM is the amalgamation of Segal's chronometry and the Standard Model (SM), a fundamental theory in particle physics. The potential applications of MLM in proton therapy are predicated on the concept of the infinite-dimensional space denoted as F_p, encompassing the entirety of proton wave functions. The inherent properties of F_p-elements f are outlined. This analysis then proceeds to capture distinct instances ("snap shot photos") of these functions at the temporal instant $t = 0$. The corresponding graphical representations of these functions are elucidated using precise geometric terminology. Specifically, two distinct types of graphs are identified: ND) a bell-shaped surface lacking a central depression, and WD) a bell-shaped surface featuring a central dent. In an endeavor to establish a connection between these mathematical revelations and proton therapy dosimetry, the exploration delves into a comparison of various classes of functions f from F_p with those produced within diverse proton therapy vaults. This integration proposes the incorporation of a novel ingredient into dosimetry, namely, the incorporation of the proton's wave function. This innovative approach holds promise for refining proton therapy techniques and enhancing treatment precision.

Keywords: proton as an elementary particle, standard and multi-level models, Wigner-Segal method, chronometric proton's space of wave functions, wave function applications to proton therapy dosimetry

1. Introduction

In accordance with the tenets of the Standard Model (SM), a proton p is postulated to consist of two u-quarks and one d-quark. Experimental evidence, particularly the detection of three distinct point-like centers through highly inelastic electron-proton scattering [1], substantiates this structural characterization of the proton. To elaborate on quark-gluon interactions, the Multi-Level Model (MLM) was introduced in Ref. [2]. Although Refs. [2, 3] have defined MLM-gluons, no subsequent developments have been pursued in this direction, making a discussion of gluons superfluous for our present topic. However, it is relevant to recall a fundamental conjecture derived from Refs. [2, 3]: (1) Free gluons manifest as detectable photons. An analogous conjecture pertaining to quarks is posited [2, 3]: (2) Free quarks materialize as protons (or antiprotons). Regarding the latter, this chapter aims to present a robust theoretical foundation, as demonstrated below in a significant portion of our content. Our treatment of the well-known SM-quarks is outlined in Section 3.

The core focus of our chapter is the exploration of the chronometric proton— a term whose implication will be clarified. While our examination predominantly revolves around this, it is important to acknowledge the involvement of other fermions such as quarks and leptons. Our overall goal also involves establishing a more rigorous foundation for the above second conjecture. Commencing with the upcoming section, we revisit the foundational principles and terminology of MLM (largely referencing [2, 3]). In our endeavor to mathematically characterize elementary particles, we employ Segal's Chronometric Theory. Notably, Section "Indecomposable Elementary Particle Associations" in Ref. [4]—effectively summarizing Segal's findings—holds a key role, and readers are advised to have this concise 5-page paper accessible as we delve into Chronometry-related aspects. The approach presented in Refs. [4] can be perceived as a generalization of Wigner's proposal [5] to model particles through specific representations of the Poincaré group, denoted as P. Intriguingly, Segal [4] delves into specific representations of G = SU(2,2), often referred to as the conformal Lie group. This group is characterized by the 4 by 4 diagonal matrix S with entries 1, 1, −1, −1. The group G encompasses 4 by 4 matrices g (with complex entries) satisfying both a determinant one condition and the equation

$$g^* Sg = S, \tag{1}$$

where g^* is the transpose and complex conjugate of g. G encompasses the extended (by scaling) Poincaré group P+ and its subgroup P, which are both 11-dimensional and 10-dimensional, respectively. The essence of Chronometry is deeply rooted in the (acclaimed!) linear-fractional G-action on the unitary group U(2), elucidated in Appendix A. For a comprehensive understanding of Segal's compact cosmos D, readers are directed to the inception of Section 2. Notably, the universal cover of D is fundamentally linked to the (renowned!) Einstein's static universe, with its three-space representation encapsulated by SU(2). In Ref. [6], the approach introduced in Ref. [4] was coined as the Wigner-Segal method, propounding a unique methodology to model elementary particles.

Overall, this introduction sets the stage for our comprehensive exploration, encompassing the SM, MLM, and Chronometry, as we endeavor to elucidate the intricate fabric of elementary particle dynamics.

In Refs. [2, 3], the MLM was introduced as a potential alternative to the SM. After further investigation (see [6–12]), it has become evident that the MLM can now be understood as a fusion of Segal's chronometry with the SM. The term "chronometric" highlights our engagement with chronometry (with its 15-dimensional core symmetry group G, as mentioned earlier). It is worth comparing the particles proposed by this theory with their relativistic counterparts, where the central symmetry group is the (10-dimensional) Poincaré group P—a fundamental player in relativistic physics. Just a reminder, the SM primarily addresses relativistic particles. In Ref. [3] (Section 2), there is a discussion of how certain traits of a chronometric particle can be interpreted within the context of relativity.

The chronometric proton p is elemental and unbreakable (so confinement is not a concern). We are fully aware that this assertion might ruffle feathers among many in the Physics community. Nevertheless, the MLM does not discard quarks entirely.

Specifically, in Refs. [2, 3], for each U(n) level where n > 2, the MLM-quark (with a specific flavor and color) was defined as a structured trio (D_{pq}, G_{ij}, m). Here, m can be either 1 or $-$ 1, depending on whether it is a particle or an antiparticle. The subgroup D_{pq} within U(n) determines flavor, while the subgroup G_{ij} within SU(n,n) determines color. An implicit aspect of this definition involves a clearly defined representation space H, where the quark's wave function finds its home. The governing group G_{ij} operates within this space.

The above paragraph has been extracted from the heart of Section 3 (sandwiched between Propositions 2 and 3) and placed here in the Introduction to offer a glimpse of what is to come for curious readers. But there is more: We interpret each MLM-quark q as a "captured proton," and q's electric charge can be either 1 or $-$ 1. Now, what about the widely accepted fractional electric charges of SM-quarks? We see this as more of an artifact—a somewhat misleading or perplexing interpretation of data.

Speaking of the representation space H mentioned earlier, it is intricately defined by the comprehensive collection F_p of chronometric proton's theoretically possible wave functions. This F_p was established in Ref. [11] and is discussed across Sections 2 (toward the end), 3, and 4.

2. From chronometry to the MLM-quarks of the U(3)-level

Mathematically, chronometry deals with a slightly larger totality of space–time events than the Minkowski space–time M has. Namely, the *compact chronometric world* D (or the *Segal's compact cosmos*), as a manifold, is the unitary group U(2). This group is defined as the totality of all two-by-two matrices z (with complex entries allowed) satisfying

$$z^* z = 1, \tag{2}$$

where 1 is the unit matrix. Here (and on), we use *world* as a synonym of *space–time*. For our purposes, it suffices to stay with U(2), which is a compact manifold. To eliminate closed time-like loops, which are unavoidable when the world is compact, one has to move to the universal covering. It is well known that D is a natural alternative of M, the unique four-dimensional manifold with comparable properties of causality and symmetry. Free particles are considered to be associated with positive-energy representations in bundles of prescribed spin over D of the group of causality-preserving transformations and with corresponding wave equations.

The imbedding of M into D *via* the Cayley transform is well known, see formula (5.2) of [13]. The Lorentzian metric (or inner product) in D was introduced by Segal (and is given in Section 3.1 of [13]). This metric is left-invariant as well as right-invariant on the Lie group U(2). It is the authors' strong belief that for the adequate understanding of the chapter, there is no need to explicitly write down this metric here. Recall that the above mentioned Poincare group P is the totality of all isometries of the (pseudo-Euclidian) M.

The main group of (causal) transformations in D is G = SU(2,2); in our Appendix A, we choose a generic element g_2 of SU(2,2) and we reproduce its action on a generic element z of D=U(2). It is the linear-fractional action.

When one switches to (an earlier mentioned) D's universal cover, one has also to switch from SU(2,2) to its universal cover. In this regard, we only mention that there is a canonical mathematical way of treating such a situation: when (an arbitrary group) G acts on U, then there is a canonical action of the G's universal cover on the U's universal cover. In our presentation, it is enough to stay with G = SU(2,2) and with its linear-fractional action on D.

Certain representations (see [4]) of SU(2,2) give rise to *chronometric particles*, but we notice, once and for all, that we only need to deal with just one particular representation, the *spannor* one: It is discussed below.

Other details on chronometry can be found in Section 2 of Ref. [3]. As it follows from [11], certain corrections (of what Segal claimed in [4], and what was reproduced from [4] in Section 2 of [3]) are to be made. The research [11] can be viewed as a discussion of, and supplement to, Segal's list of chronometric elementary particles of spin 1/2 [4]. The last article is in some sense a summary of Segal's findings, and it is just 5 pages long. In Ref. [4], there are few, if any, clues of how to obtain results outlined in it. In publication [11], one of the main goals was to prove (some of) Segal's statements. The most remarkable of these is that there are four elementary chronometric particles of spin 1/2. Namely, there is a massive neutral particle named the exon, the electron e, and two types of neutrino (interpreted as v_e and v_μ). The authors of Ref. [11] failed to prove that (but see what is said right below). In Segal's theory, a particle (e.g., each of the above) is mathematically associated with an irreducible unitary positive-energy representations of the symmetry group G (in our case, the conformal group SU(2; 2)). Below, we associate certain mathematical objects with specific particles; Doing so, we try to stay in line with what Segal has done before in this regard. Here is the only significant exception to the above: around 2010 A. Levichev suggested in Ref. [14], Section 7, that it is rather the proton p than a hypothetical neutral particle, the exon.

Levichev's Multi-Level Model of quarks, MLM [2, 3] claims that each SM-quark can be viewed as a "sunken (i.e., submerged) proton." From Ref. [11], there is just one neutrino, rather than two, as in Ref. [4].

An earlier conjecture by Segal (about the number of chronometric spin 1/2 particles) was in compliance with the findings in Ref. [11], see [15] (Th. 16.7.10) that worked with a 3-step composition series. The spannor representation is a limiting case of representations studied by Jakobsen in Ref. [14], where, purely algebraically, a 3-step series may be obtained after the fact. Later, Segal's original (i.e., the one of [15]) conclusion has been withdrawn: Table 1 of Ref. [4] states (without proof) the existence of the 4-step composition series. Overall, the authors of Ref. [11] follow the approach of Ref. [4]. Below (in this Section), we give more details from Ref. [11]. In the general context of how to mathematically define the notion of an elementary particle, we comment there on the transition from the renowned Wigner method to (what was called in Ref. [6] as) the Wigner–Segal method. From Ref. [11], there is a certain (infinite-dimensional) Hilbert space F_p (of functions on the Minkowski space–time M) that is interpreted as the set of all (theoretically possible) *states* (i.e., *wave functions*) of the chronometric proton p (see formula (20) of [11] and Theorem 3.1 of [10]). (More details on the space F_p are given in our Section 4.) The group G = SU (2,2) acts on F_p. According to the terminology of Ref. [10], Remark 4.1, this G is the *ruling group*, G_r, since it *rules* (or *governs*) the behavior of the particle.

As a mathematical model, MLM deals with the sequence of *canonical* (i.e., based on principal minors of the matrices involved) embeddings of groups: U(2) into U(3), U(2) into U(4), U(2) into U(5), and so forth. Each of these embeddings is an isomorphism onto the corresponding subgroup. These isomorphisms play an essential role on how to relate our MLM-quarks to the SM-quarks (for a quicker understanding of the MLM, go to Figure A1 of the Appendix A in [12]). The above groups were called *levels*: U(2) is the 0th level; U(3), the 1st; U(4), the 2nd; and so on. In Ref. [12], Section 3, it is shown that such a convention matches the standard quarks' generations' list. Recall that each matrix group U(n) is defined quite similarly to how U(2) was defined by our Eq. (2). Embeddings A_{12}, A_{13}, A_{23} of (the Segal's compact cosmos) D = U(2) into U(3) were introduced as follows: Under each of these three embeddings, a matrix Z from D becomes a certain principal 2 by 2 minor of the corresponding 3 by 3 matrix from U(3). Namely, denote by D_{12} the image of the embedding A_{12}. The A_{12}, itself, is defined right below (also, these embeddings are illustrated in the top portion of Figure A1 of the Appendix A in Ref. [12]).

Each Z from D is put as an upper 2 by 2 principal minor of the 3 by 3 matrix $A_{12}(Z)$ in U(3); the third diagonal entry of $A_{12}(Z)$ is 1; in the $A_{12}(Z)$, any other entry is zero. The two remaining embeddings, A_{13} and A_{23}, are defined quite similarly. Clearly, D_{12}, D_{13}, and D_{23} are U(2)–subgroups in U(3). Obviously, the group U(2) is closed with respect to the complex conjugation, and with respect to. the matrix transposition. The transposed matrix Z^T is obtained from Z by reflection in the principal diagonal. Hence, each of the D_{12}, D_{13}, and D_{23} is invariant with respect to any of the two mentioned operations in U(3). Also, to enumerate all D_{ij}, it is enough to consider the cases i < j, only. Each D_{ij} carries a Lorentzian metric by the demand that each A_{ij} be an isometry.

In the totality of all *m* by *m* matrices, P_m is introduced, as the symmetry with respect to the opposite diagonal. Clearly, when Z is in U(2), then $P_2(Z)$ is also in U(2). From this, it follows that the subgroup D_{13} is P_3-invariant in U(3) while $P_3(D_{12}) = D_{23}$, $P_3(D_{23}) = D_{12}$. That enables us to view the embeddings A_{12} and A_{23} as equivalent (one becomes the other when composed with P_3 and P_2—see Figure A1 of the Appendix A in [12]). This relates to the "presence of two SM-*u*-quarks in" a proton, while the A_{13} relates to the presence of an SM-*d*-quark in that proton. These embeddings make it possible to introduce a notion of a flavor of any MLM-quark of level U(3). The last two phrases are "nonmathematical;" we relate to physics here. We discuss this in more detail later in this section (right after Theorem 1).

Definition 1. Let us use the name cell for each of these D_{ij}.

It should always be stated (or should be clear from the context) which U(n)-level such a cell is considered to be in.

In Ref. [3], Section 3, similar to the way of introducing in U(3) of the U(2)-subgroups D_{12}, D_{13}, and D_{23}, the SU(2,2)-subgroups G_{12}, G_{13}, and G_{23} of SU(3,3) have been defined. In our Appendix A, G_{12} and G_{13} are presented graphically. Namely, a generic element (of each of the two subgroups) is explicitly shown there. At each level U(n), any subgroup G_{ij} is defined in Section 4 of Ref. [12] (right before Proposition 2 there)—quite similar to how it has been done for the U(3)-level.

Definition 2. Let us use the name ruling (i.e., governing) group, or the *r*-group, for each of these G_{ij} (the latter being an SU(2,2)-subgroup of SU(n,n), in general).

It should always be stated (or should be clear from the context) which U(n)-level such an *r*-group is associated with. From Ref. [6], we now reproduce the following statement.

Theorem 1. *An action of each of the subgroups* G_{12}, G_{13}, *and* G_{23} *on any of the subgroups* D_{12}, D_{13} *and* D_{23} *is defined. In particular, each of the following three actions,* G_{12} *on* D_{12}, G_{13} *on* D_{13}, *and* G_{23} *on* D_{23}, *is the linear-fractional one.*

What about the mathematical meaning (and about the physical interpretation) of the following phrase (from above): "The embeddings A_{12} and A_{23} relate to the presence of two SM-*u*-quarks in a proton, while the A_{13} relates to the presence of an SM-*d*-quark in that proton"?

According to the SM, a proton consists of two *u*-quarks and of one *d*-quark. The detection of three point-like centers (of highly inelastic electron-proton scattering, see [1]) served as an experimental basis for such a conclusion about the structure of a proton. However, after several decades of intense search, the majority of the Physics community has submitted to the view that "free quarks cannot be detected."

Above, we have been discussing chronometric particles of spin ½. They originate from an induced representation of the group G = SU(2,2) defined by formula (5) from Section 2 of Ref. [11]. In Ref. [11], three chronometric spin ½ fermions have been mathematically detected: proton *p*, electronic neutrino v_e, and electron *e*. On the basis of formula (16) from Ref. [11], the space F of the induced representation (sometimes referred to as the *spannor representation*, see [16]) of the group G = SU(2,2) has been introduced. In F, there exist two nontrivial invariant subspaces with no invariant complement. One of those subspaces was denoted by F_p, and it was supplied with a Hilbert space structure. On the basis of the findings in Refs. [17, 18], the following statement has been proven (see Section 5 of [11]):

Theorem 2. *The restriction of the induced representation to* F_p *is unitary and irreducible. In* F_p, *the energy-positivity condition holds.*

The space F_p has been interpreted as the totality of all (theoretically possible) wave functions of the chronometric proton. Notice that F_p is of *conformal weight* (or *conformal dimension*) 5/2, see Ref. [11].

Remark 1. Let us repeat that in Ref. [11], it was stated that F_p does not have an invariant complement. It means that we deal with the case where the Wigner method is not applicable. According to the Wigner-Segal method, introduce the quotient space $W = F/F_p$ and the factor-representation in it. In Section 6 of Ref. [11], a minimal nontrivial invariant subspace F_v in W has been supplied with the unitary structure and it has been interpreted as the totality of all wave functions of the chronometric electronic neutrino. In Ref. [11], Section 7, the quotient space $W/F_v = F_e$ has been interpreted as the totality of all wave functions of the chronometric electron (since the corresponding factor-representation turned out to be irreducible and unitarizable, and the conformal weight is 3/2 now). This was the final step in the proof of the main finding of Ref. [11]: There are exactly three elementary chronometric spin 1/2 particles.

Remark 2. Having in mind Remark 9.1 of Ref. [11], from now on, it seems plausible to associate the Hilbert space F_v with the electronic antineutrino, rather than with electronic neutrino. The authors of Ref. [11] followed Segal (see [4]), and they interpreted this ("middle") sector of the 3-step composition series as the one corresponding to the electronic neutrino, but (also in [11]) they have envisaged a possibility of the antineutrino interpretation. Such an interpretation can serve as a mathematical reason allowing a return (as it has been claimed in [19]) to an "old model" for the neutron as consisting of a proton, of an electron, and of an electronic antineutrino—see the U(2)-part of the Figure A4 (in the Appendix A of [12]).

For the level U(3), clearly, each A_{ij} is an isometry, and each D_{ij} is a space–time isometric to the Segal's compact cosmos D. From here (and on the basis of both the above Theorem 2 and of its interpretation), we conclude that a spin ½ fermion ("living in" D_{ij}) is mathematically defined. If D_{12} or D_{23} is a support of its wave functions, then, as part of the MLM-settings, we associate this fermion with an *u*-quark. If D_{13} is such a support, then the particle is interpreted as a *d*-quark. It means that in the MLM, we have introduced two flavors for quarks of the 1st level, U(3), and (by merely keeping the SM-terminology) we have established the correspondence of MLM-quarks to the SM-quarks, and vice versa. The Hilbert structure in the corresponding spaces H_{ij} is introduced *via* the isometries A_{ij} from the original H = F_p. For each of our fermions of the level U(3), its ruling group G can be any of G_{12}, G_{13}, or G_{23}. Such a convention was a mathematical basis for defining the notion of a *color* of an MLM-quark (see Sections 3 and 4 of [6], as well as our Section 3, below). Clearly, each MLM-quark is as fully described as the chronometric proton was—see our Theorem 2, above. We are thus able to interpret each MLM-quark q as a "captured proton": a certain G_{ij} is its ruling group and q stays within the U(3) level.

Back to the highly inelastic electron-proton scattering: as the result of it, proton gets (from U(2)) to a "deeper" level, U(3). In U(3), it gets to one particular cell (of the total of three available ones: D_{12}, D_{13}, or D_{23}), thus "becoming an MLM-quark". In terms of Physics, a possible description (see our Section 3, below) could use the following wording: our proton pushes "deeper" (i.e., to the U(4)-level) the "former occupant" of this cell. However, to better understand such a wording, one has to read our Section 3 first.

Since Ref. [12] has introduced equivalence (w.r.t. operators P_3 and P_2—see Figure A1 of the Appendix A there) between D_{12} and D_{23}, we only have two flavors rather than three. In a formal agreement with the SM, our description of the highly inelastic scattering is that of the elastic one, but on quarks (in our case, on MLM-quarks). In particular, within the U(3) level, we should use another Hilbert space and another *r*-group.

Figures B1–B4 (of our Appendix B) show what specific geometric properties a proton's wave function might have (= "what our proton might look like"). Seemingly, the thus suggested description of the highly inelastic electron-proton scattering does not, per se, contradict to detection, [1], of "three point-like components in a proton." Also, in the MLM-approach, one can directly apply the combinatorial SM-methods to calculate relations between certain scattering probabilities. As an example ([12], p. 6), it is demonstrated that the ratio of (full) cross sections between πp- and pp-scatterings is in compliance with the SM-approach (while the latter fits experimental findings). Since (below) we discuss the "*submerged* vs. *captured*" proton, let us mention that **Figures B1–B3** are indicative of the case of a captured proton while **Figure B4** is of the submerged one.

3. An overview of the SM-quarks' generations and the introduction of the MLM-quarks at "deeper" levels

Let us continue with more MLM-details. If our proton gets into the cell D_{12}, then we have to exploit the space F_{12} of wave functions defined on D_{12}, rather than on the original D. Due to the isometry A_{12} between D and D_{12}, the Hilbert spaces F_p and F_{12} are unitarily equivalent. In Ref. [6], the notation $q(1;1,2)$ has been used for such an

MLM-quark: the first "1" is the level number (i.e., the U(3) level), while the pair (1,2) specifies the cell as D_{12}. Denoting the embeddings of D=U(2) into U(4) as A_{12}, A_{13}, A_{14}, A_{23}, A_{24}, and A_{34} (see Figure A2 of Appendix A in [12]), the notation mimics the one already used in the U(3)-case. To determine equivalences, consider the operator P_4: the symmetry with respect to the opposite diagonal. Clearly (as Figure A2 of [12] illustrates), A_{12} is equivalent to A_{34}, and A_{13} is equivalent to A_{24}. Each of the subgroups D_{14} and D_{23} is P_4-invariant. Relate A_{14} to an SM-quark s and A_{23} to an SM-quark c. At this (i.e., at the second) level, A_{12} (which is equivalent to A_{34}) relates to an SM-quark u, while A_{13} (equivalent to A_{24}) relates to an SM-quark d. Hence, SM-quarks of both *generations* (one and two) "live" on the 2nd MLM-level, U(4).

Now, proceed with an overview of the SM-quarks' generations, as well as of the topic in general. According to http://phys.vspu.ac.ru/forstudents/TSOR/Kutseva/pokolenie_leptonov_i_kvarkov.html, by 2018, it was known that there exist (at least) three generations of quarks and three generations of leptons. These fundamental particles are thought to be adequately modeled as the "point-like" ones. Both quarks and leptons have spin ½, which means that they are fermions. By convention, a *fermion* is a particle with half-integer spin, while a *boson* is a particle with an integer spin. Mathematically, a spin of a particle is a certain constant that is present in the (describing this very particle) representation of the group G—see, for instance, p. 348 of Ref. [20]. By G here (as well as above), we mean the main group of transformations acting in the space–time that our particle "lives in." The word *generation* is part of the SM-terminology; generations will be naturally "built into" the MLM—see below. For other necessary details about fermions and of their role as seen by the SM, see Section 3 of [12]. The MLM-description of higher (than U(4)) level quarks is also given in that Section 3. From there, we only reproduce the following.

Remark 3. The SM-quarks of higher generations were detected later than SM-quarks of lower generations: with the increase of the accelerators' typical energies. Hence, it is natural to interpret the "deepening,", as n gets larger, of the U(n)-levels as corresponding to the increase of the scattering typical energy.

From [2, 3], reproduce Theorem 3.

Theorem 3. *On the level* U(n), *suppose an* U(2)-*subgroup* D_{ij} *be not* P_n-*invariant. Then,* D_{ij} *corresponds to a quark from a lower level. The recurrent (3) and explicit (4) formulas (for the total number* m_n *of quarks at the* U(n)-*level) hold:*

$$m_2 = 1, m_n = m_{n-1} + [n/2], \tag{3}$$

$$m_n = \{n(n-1)/2 + [n/2]\}/2. \tag{4}$$

Here, [x] denotes the greatest integer part ("roof") of a real number x. We are thankful to the reviewer of [12] who has noticed that (4) can be simply expressed as $[n^2/4]$.

The "selection criterion" (i.e., why are we quite satisfied with our list of MLM-quarks) is the one that establishes their explicit correspondence with the SM-quarks. In levels U(3), U(4), and U(5), the MLM-quarks are in precise correspondence with the SM-quarks as they are currently agreed upon. In level U(6), three new SM-quarks are predicted, as illustrated by Figure A3 [12].

On p. 8 of Ref. [12], right after Remark 5 there, the color of an MLM-quark D_{sk} was defined as G_{ij} (which can be chosen from G_{12}, G_{13}, G_{23}). In other words, the color of an MLM-quark is defined by the choice of its ruling group (or, even more formally, the color (as a symbol) of an MLM-quark is (the symbol of) its ruling group). Recall that the ruling group also acts in the Hilbert space of wave functions of the quark in question (compared to what we have stated earlier, right after Remark 2). Clearly, there are three colors for quarks of the U(3)-level.

Now, let us introduce the notion of a color for an arbitrary U(n), with the integer n no less than 3. Given an embedding A_{ij} of $D = U(2)$ into $U(n)$, by G_{ij}, we understand a certain, uniquely defined SU(2,2)-subgroup in $G_n = SU(n,n)$. Namely, G_{ij} consists of certain matrices g_n, uniquely defined by four n by n blocks A_n, B_n, C_n, and D_n. These four blocks are uniquely defined by the matrix g_2 (chosen arbitrarily) from $G_2 = SU$ (2,2); in particular, G_{ij} is isomorphic to SU(2,2)—see Proposition 2, below. To continue, g_2 is determined by its 2 by 2 blocks A_2, B_2, C_2, D_2. To define n by n blocks A_n, B_n, C_n, D_n for g_n, proceed as follows (also, see our Appendix A). The block A_n is defined according to (1) and (2): (1) A_2 is that very minor in A_n; (2) any other entry in A_n is 1 (if on the principal diagonal) or it is zero (if it is off the principal diagonal)—compared to how G_{12} was defined in our Section 2. The block D_n is defined quite similarly but with the help of D_2. The two remaining blocks, B_n and C_n, are defined (in terms of B_2 and C_2) somewhat differently. Namely, each entry, which is off the corresponding 2 by 2 principal minor of the block, is zero. The following statement has been proven in Ref. [3].

Proposition 2. G_{ij} is a subgroup of G_n; G_{ij} is isomorphic to SU(2,2).

In Refs. [2, 3], for each level U(n), with n greater than 2, the MLM-quark (of a certain flavor and color) was defined as an ordered triple (D_{pq}, G_{ij}, m). Here m is either 1 or negative 1 (depending on whether we deal with a particle or with an antiparticle). The subgroup D_{pq} in U(n) determines flavor, while the subgroup G_{ij} in SU(n,n) determines color. An implicit part of this definition is a well-defined representation space H, which the quark's wave function belongs to. The ruling (i.e., governing) group G_{ij} acts in this H.

The following statement has been proven in Ref. [3]:

Proposition 3. The total number of colors at the U(n)-level is n(n-1)/2.

According to the SM (with its total number of colors being 3), the electric charge of each quark u (or c, or t) is 2/3, while the electric charge of each quark d (or s, or b) is minus 1/3. There is an approach with integer quarks' electric charges [21]. Such an approach is known as the Han-Nambu scheme (in [21], there is a reference to the original Han-Nambu publications). Part of the Section 4 (in [12]) deals with an adaptation of the Han-Nambu scheme to the MLM.

Starting with the U(3)-level, here is the following possible interpretation in terms of physics: when a proton (participating in highly inelastic scattering) "finds itself" in a D_{13}-cell (and it stays there for a moment, name it a *submerged proton*), then its color may be one of G_{12}, G_{23}, or G_{13} but changing between them with huge speed, presumably. A. Levichev likes a comparison with a "hot potato scenario" here: It is hardly possible to hold a hot potato in just one hand! Substitute "potato" by "proton" and "a hand" by "a ruling group." The total number of ruling groups of the level U(n) increases as n gets larger. As stated in the Table 1 of Ref. [12], in D_{13}, these ruling subgroups generate electric charges 0, 0, negative 1, in that order. It means that a quark d has an average charge of negative 1/3. Similarly, a u-quark has charge 2/3. Notice that (from now on), we use *submerged* instead of *sank* (which appeared in [3]). As regards an *electric charge generated by the ruling group*, more details are provided in subsection 6.2 of [12].

On the basis of our Remark 2, above, and of the suggested MLM- approach to the values of SM-quarks' electric charges, the following conjecture is logically noncontradictory:

Conjecture 1. The electric charges of the proton and of the electron (both viewed either "inside" neutron, or separately) originate as the result of the corresponding action (in their Hilbert spaces F_p and F_e) of the ruling group G (represented, essentially, by SU(2,2)).

This ("philosophical") view might serve as an answer (preliminary, at least) to the question "What are the origins of electric charge?" According to the SM (as well as to the MLM), there are color charges, too. Is it possible to interpret the chronometric proton's electric charge as a special case of the MLM-quarks' color charges? In the U(2)-level, there is just one ruling group for the proton, which means that there is just one color. Can we interpret this color charge as the electric charge of the chronometric proton?

The number of colors (in a given MLM-level) is level-dependent (see Proposition 3, above). In the U(5)-level, the electric charge values of MLM-quarks (in the "sunken proton" situation) are (slightly) different from those of the corresponding SM-quarks—see ([12], Section 4). Clearly, detection of this discrepancy might be a challenge for the current experimental physics!

In Section 5 of Ref. [12], the compilation of fermion triplets across levels U(2) through U(5) offers valuable insights into the potential structure of matter at deeper MLM-levels. Could the detection of hadron jets possibly serve as an indicator of this intriguing "MLM-structure"? It is plausible that this structure could undergo local disruptions during high-energy interactions, providing a more reasonable explanation than those proposed by the Standard Model. In this context, A. Levichev recollects his astonishment while navigating through PDG-files (available at http://pdg.lbl.gov/2018/reviews/rpp2018-rev-structure-functions.pdf). In Section 18.4, he encountered the term "hadronic structure of the photon," a phrase that left a lasting impact. It is his aspiration that within scientific and medical circles, the prevailing perspective would lean toward regarding both photons and protons as elementary particles.

Concluding this section, we offer additional MLM-related insights, some in support, while others point out specific challenges and potential directions for future research.

Remark 4. The chronometric interactions are mathematically classified by Segal in Ref. ([4], p. 996). Before we implement his findings into the MLM-scheme, we need to double-check the constituents of the chronometric bosonic sector. As regards the MLM-Lagrangian, the challenges "hide" in the chronometry, already. Here is what Segal ([4], p. 995) said in this regard: "The elementary particles in chronometric theory are closely integrated into coherent entities ... ", he calls them clans, " ... Scalar, spinor, and vector elementary particles arise as subunits, and the fundamental interaction is between fermion and boson clans as entities, the total interaction Lagrangian being representable as a sum of interactions between individual elementary particles only in the relativistic limit." The (mathematically pretty "delicate") notion of the *conformal weight* plays the key role in classifying fundamental chronometric interactions: ([4], pp. 996, 997). As it has been detected in Ref. [11], the chronometric neutrino is not a particle of a certain conformal weight. This puts us in front of a new challenge: one has to modify, at least, the just mentioned Segal's classification of chronometric interactions.

Figure A3 in Ref. [12] illustrates the MLM's U(6)-level, and it suggests "where" to search for the (three) SM-quarks of the 4th generation—another challenge for the SM-experimental quest.

Overall, to the key MLM-conjecture, [12], that "an SM-quark can be interpreted either as a sunken or as a captured proton," our chapter provides additional arguments. Unfortunately, we are not yet in a position to better support a claim of [3]—"At each level, a gluon can be interpreted as a colored and flavored photon," since in order to do that, we have to start with a check of the bosonic sector findings by Segal. Recall that in Ref. [11], a similar check has been performed for the fermionic sector. Nevertheless, even at this point in time, it seems appropriate to mention the following chronometric findings: the key bosons (photon γ, W-boson, Z-boson) have been mathematically detected [4]. As regards the Higgs boson, on p. 996 of [4], Segal indicates the absence of one. To our mind (due to what we have above said), the Higgs boson existence stays as an open (mathematical) MLM-question, so far.

4. On the proton's wave function and on its real-valued analogue

So far, the proton's wave function in the literature (which we have had a look at) was treated in terms of proton's quark constituents, like in https://physics.stack exchange.com/questions/2786/visualization-of-protons-wavefunction and in https://www.physicsforums.com/threads/do-protons-and-neutrons-have-a-wavefunc tions.243322/.

Our view on proton is different, see the Introduction where the totality of its wave functions has been denoted as F_p and later, in Section 2 (Theorem 2), main properties of F_p have been stated. Right now, we provide more details on F_p.

In Ref. [11], the Minkowski space–time M is represented as a certain set of 2 by 2 matrices; let us use **h** to denote such an element (= *event*) in M:

$$\mathbf{h} = \begin{bmatrix} x_0 + x_1 & x_2 + ix_3 \\ x_2 - ix_3 & x_0 - x_1 \end{bmatrix}. \tag{5}$$

In (5), above, real numbers x_0, x_1, x_2, x_3 are (standard) coordinates of the event in question; we say *standard*, meaning the case when M is presented as a four-dimensional vector space with a Lorentzian metric. It follows from Ref. ([11], eq. (20)) that each value of the proton's wave function Ψ at **h** is the following vector in a complex 2-dimensional linear space C^2:

$$\Psi[\mathbf{w}, \mathbf{v}](\mathbf{h}) = K(\mathbf{h}, \mathbf{w})\mathbf{v} \tag{6}$$

By w^*, below, we denote the matrix obtained from **w** by transposition and complex conjugation; **w**, above, belongs to a certain class of 2 by 2 matrices (see [11], Section 4). In the above (6), the notation $\Psi[\mathbf{w},\mathbf{v}]$ presumes that the wave function is defined as soon as the parameters **w** and **v** are chosen; here, **v** is from C^2. Also, the *reproducing kernel K* in (6) is defined by

$$K(\mathbf{w}_1, \mathbf{w}_2) = \{(\mathbf{w}_1 - \mathbf{w}_2{}^*)/(2i)\}^{-1}\left\{\det\left[\{(\mathbf{w}_1 - \mathbf{w}_2{}^*)/(2i)\}^{-2}\right.\right., \tag{7}$$

where $\mathbf{w}_1$, $\mathbf{w}_2$ are taken from the abovementioned class of 2 by 2 matrices. It is well-known that expression (7) is always mathematically meaningful.

Essentially, we have thus introduced an (infinite-dimensional) Hilbert space F_p (of functions on the Minkowski space–time M), which is interpreted as the set of all (theoretically possible) *states* (or *wave functions*) of the chronometric proton p. This F_p

is the completion of the span of the set of functions (6). The positive definite inner product $<.,.>$ in F_p is defined as follows:

$$<\Psi_1, \Psi_2> \ = \ <K(w_1, w_2)v_1, v_2>, \qquad (8)$$

where, in the right side of (8), the canonical inner product in C^2 is meant. As it has been stated in our Theorem 2, the restriction of the induced representation to F_p is unitary and irreducible. Here, the Mackey's concept of induced representation is meant. This concept proved to be a major tool in the modern quantum mechanical description of a particle (see [20]). We apologize to the reader that the abovementioned representation (which is known as the *spannor representation* [4, 16]) cannot be fully described in our current text. We only recall that it is induced from a certain finite-dimensional representation of the (extended by scaling, and thus being 11-dimensional) Poincare group.

Using eq. (15) of [11], we have:

$$L(h) = SAv, \qquad (9)$$

with always defined

$$S = \{\det [(h{-}w)/(2i)]\}^{-2}. \qquad (10)$$

Introduce the (real-valued!) function f as follows:

$$f(h) = L^*L, \qquad (11)$$

where (for brevity) in the right side, we omit the argument h. To word it differently, the value of f at h is the Hermitian square of the vector in the right side of (6). From now, and till the end of Section 4, we refer to (11) as to the proton's wave function. The expression for the 2 by 2 matrix A is (reproduced from [22]) as follows:

$$A = 2i(h{-}w^*)^{-1}. \qquad (12)$$

In publication [22], the entries in (5), (9), and (10) have been specified as follows: $x_0 = x_1 = 0$; components of vector v: $v_1 = 0$, $v_2 = 1$; $w = \begin{bmatrix} 1+i & -1 \\ -1 & 1+i \end{bmatrix}$. This results in $h = \begin{bmatrix} 0 & z \\ \bar{z} & 0 \end{bmatrix}$ with $z = x + iy$. It means that in (5), we have simplified x_2 to x and x_3 to y. In our Appendix B, we thus deal with the real-valued function f(x,y). Here, x and y are the "usual" coordinates on the plane, while the remaining two coordinates (time t and the third space coordinate) are chosen as 0. In other words, it is the case of a "toy proton"; it was a first try (see [22]) to understand what kind of functions might be there, in the proton's Hilbert space F_p. Dropping a (positive) constant factor, we end up with $f(x,y) = ((x + 1)^2 + y^2 + 2)\lambda^{-3}$ where $\lambda = ((x + 1)^2 + y^2)^2 + 4$. It turns out that f(x,y) has just one local minimum, at $(-1,0)$ as shown on **Figure B1**. The totality of all points where f(x,y) reaches its maximum V is a circle defined by the equation $(x + 1)^2 + y^2 = r^2$. The radius r of this circle is determined from the system of equations for critical points of f(x,y). The highest points of the graph (as shown on **Figures B2** and **B3**) form a circle that lies in the U = V plane; here, U is for the third coordinate in 3-space where we plot (portions of) the graph of f(x,y). The findings are graphically presented: **Figures B1–B3**. It is a *bell-shaped* surface *with a dent on top*. Clearly, it is important to move from this toy example to a more realistic one where f depends on all three space variables—we will refer to this case as to a "realistic proton," see below. Notice that, obviously, f(**h**) in (11) is positive. We continue to refer to such an f(**h**) as to the "proton's wave function" (despite a formal contradiction of (11) with formula (6), from above)—compared to how we have put it in Section 4 title: *its real-valued analogue*. When we allow for the third spatial dimension z, staying with the same **v** and with the same **w**, the result is as follows.

Theorem 4. *The resulting proton's wave function is given by*

$$f(x, y, z) = \left((x+1)^2 + y^2 + (z-1)^2 + 1\right)\lambda^{-3}, \tag{13}$$

where $\lambda = ((x + 1)^2 + y^2 + z^2)^2 + 4$. *As a 3-dimensional surface in* R^4 *(with a 'vertical' coordinate U), the graph*

$$U = f(x, y, z), \tag{14}$$

is a bell-shaped surface E *(with no dent on top). The highest point of* E *corresponds to the input* $(-1,0,z_1)$ *where* z_1 *is the (only!) real root of* $5z^5 - 11z^4 + 12z^3 - 4z + 4 = 0$. *Numerically,* z_1 *is close to negative 0.65. The point* $(-1,0,z_1)$ *is the center of our (realistic) proton.*

Remark 5. Due to the chapter space limitation, we are unable to present all the details of the Theorem 4 proof. The plot of E's typical section by a "vertical" 3-plane through the highest point of E is given by **Figure B4**. Not all cuts of E by U = const 3-planes are spheres (compared to a "toy proton" wave function where all of its graph cuts by horizontal 2-planes were circles).

Clearly, when z = 0 is entered into (13), we get our f(x,y), from above. That is, when we cut E by z = 0 3-plane, the result is a bell-shaped 2-surface with a dent on top.

Consider the following function:

$$g(x, y, z) = \left((x+1)^2 + y^2 + z^2 + 2\right)\lambda^{-3}, \tag{15}$$

with $\lambda = ((x + 1)^2 + y^2 + z^2)^2 + 4$. Here is the equation of its graph J with such a ("desired") spherical symmetry (w.r.t. the cuts by U = const 3-planes) property:

$$U = g(x, y, z). \tag{16}$$

Obviously, the cut of J by the z = 0 3-plane is exactly the 2-dimensional surface shown on **Figures B1–B3**. It is so, since the input of z = 0 into (15) results in f(x,y) for the "toy proton", from above.

Also, it is not difficult to show that J is a bell-shaped surface with a dent on top. Does g(x,y,z) originate from an element of F_p *via* formula (11)? It is an open question, so far.

5. Conclusion

As highlighted in the Introduction, the logical sequence of this chapter unfolds as follows. Our foundational cornerstone, serving as both our starting point and robust theoretical basis, is the MLM-theory, at times referred to as a fusion of Segal's chronometry with the Standard Model. From the MLM perspective, protons emerge as the fundamental elementary particles of the natural world, supplanting the prominence of SM-quarks. This audacious assertion naturally necessitates a broader inclusion of mathematical descriptions for other essential particles, recognizing the significance of interactions in the grand scheme. In Sections 1 through 3, we establish essential mathematical frameworks and concepts, subsequently delving into a multitude of MLM-related applications and interpretations within the realm of Physics. All these endeavors have been distilled succinctly, with the intention to persuade the reader that a proton, in isolation, can, from the MLM standpoint, encompass the ability to model every current physical phenomenon explained through SM-quarks. Our modeling framework introduces novel concepts, including the notions of a sunken or submerged ("pritoplennyi" in Russian) proton, a captured proton, and the concept of the ruling group.

Only after we have navigated through a range of specific MLM-discoveries and challenges from a panoramic theoretical stance (particularly evident starting from Conjecture 1 and continuing through the culmination of Section 3), do we find ourselves suitably poised to revisit the crux of the matter—the chronometric proton itself. In Section 4, we dive deeper into the intricacies of F_p, the aggregate of its wave functions. While earlier, in Section 2 (Theorem 2), we established fundamental properties of F_p, our primary aim in Section 4 was to capture a snapshot of the proton's wave function at the temporal juncture $t = 0$ and subsequently elucidate its corresponding graph through precise geometric terms. In a partial success (refer to Section 4 for comprehensive details), it appears we have managed to discern at least two distinct types of graphs, reflective of "members" within F_p: A) ND-case, a bell-shaped curve without a dent at its peak, and B) WD-case, a bell-shaped curve featuring a central dent. It is tentatively proposed that the ND-case corresponds to a submerged proton, while the WD-case corresponds to a captured proton, influenced by a specific ruling group.

While our journey to connect these findings with proton therapy dosimetry is still a work in progress, it is important to acknowledge the timeline of our key papers—[11, 12, 22]—which were recently published in 2022. We anticipate a surge of research contributions on this topic, especially after the publication of this book featuring our chapter. Moving forward, we outline potential avenues of exploration in the subsequent section, marking out the trajectories for future research endeavors.

6. Could our discoveries find relevance in the domain of proton therapy dosimetry?

Admittedly, it might seem a stretch to envision a direct application of our deeply theoretical and mathematically intricate proton description to practical medical contexts. Nevertheless, let us contemplate this within the realm of proton therapy.

Throughout our chapter, spanning from its inception and threading through the theoretical exposition of the chronometric proton, and further into Section 4 with its specific revelations, the spotlight remains firmly on the concept of the wave function. However, the question of whether the wave function possesses a tangible existence and what it truly signifies continues to loom large within the framework of quantum mechanics. This quandary has bewildered many prominent physicists, in the past and present. Notably, a substantial contingent of experts—though perhaps not the dominant majority—aligns with our standpoint: that the wave function must indeed possess an objective and physical reality. This perspective opens the door to exploring correlations between our findings and distinct designs of proton vaults.

Consider the scenario where diverse proton vaults give rise to proton beams of varying configurations. Within this context, our focus narrows in on the intriguing prospect of classifying these beams and subsequently linking them to distinctive characteristics of the proton's wave function. Unfortunately, this promising avenue of research, aimed at applying our insights to proton therapy dosimetry—the discipline concerned with measuring, computing, and evaluating absorbed radiation doses (see [23, 24])—came into our purview relatively late. The constraints of the present chapter prevent an exhaustive exploration of this direction.

Yet it is conceivable that the notion of the proton's wave function has remained untapped in studies comparing different proton vaults. We posit that the prevailing understanding of "similar proton beam configurations" does not preclude differences among protons (within two ostensibly similar beams) based on their respective wave functions—a discovery we unveiled in Section 4. Moreover, it is important to note that the scope extends beyond the two cases we addressed in Section 4 and mentioned in Section 5, such as the ND-case and the WD-case. For instance, even two surfaces each devoid of a dent on top might exhibit disparities in terms of the sharpness or spread of their peaks.

The potential implications of our research extend into the clinical realm. As ongoing proton therapy clinical trials amass substantial statistical data, our ongoing contemplations will be put to the test through robust experimental validation. This accumulation of empirical evidence holds the promise of yielding definitive pro/con assessments. Intriguingly, a different perspective could also shed light on the perplexing "reality of the wave function" enigma. Should similar configurations of proton beams—when applied in comparable clinical scenarios—yield divergent outcomes, it could serve as an indirect pointer toward an affirmative resolution to this longstanding puzzle.

In essence, our exploration serves as a catalyst for new inquiries within the domain of proton therapy, potentially ushering in a novel era where the intricate interplay between wave functions and proton configurations contributes to both practical applications and the deeper understanding of fundamental quantum concepts.

Acknowledgements

The research by A. Levichev was partly funded by the State Program of fundamental scientific research of the Sobolev Institute of Mathematics (SB RAS, project No FWNF-2022-0006). The research by M. Neshchadim was partly funded by the State Program of fundamental scientific research of the Sobolev Institute of Mathematics (SB RAS, project No FWNF-2022-0009).

Appendix A (i.e., graphic details on ruling groups)

$$g_{12} = \begin{bmatrix} A & 0 & B & 0 \\ 0 & 1 & 0 & 0 \\ C & 0 & D & 0 \\ 0 & 0 & 0 & 1 \end{bmatrix}, g_{13} = \begin{bmatrix} A_1 & 0 & A_2 & B_1 & 0 & B_2 \\ 0 & 1 & 0 & 0 & 0 & 0 \\ A_3 & 0 & A_4 & B_3 & 0 & B_4 \\ C_1 & 0 & C_2 & D_1 & 0 & D_2 \\ 0 & 0 & 0 & 0 & 1 & 0 \\ C_3 & 0 & C_4 & D_3 & 0 & D_4 \end{bmatrix}, \qquad (17)$$

where in case of g_{12}, the 4 by 4 matrix g_2 was denoted as $\begin{bmatrix} A & B \\ C & D \end{bmatrix}$, while in case of g_{13}, the 4 by 4 matrix g_2 was also denoted as $\begin{bmatrix} A & B \\ C & D \end{bmatrix}$, but with further specification of its 2 by 2 blocks: $A = \begin{bmatrix} A_1 & A_2 \\ A_3 & A_4 \end{bmatrix}, B = \begin{bmatrix} B_1 & B_2 \\ B_3 & B_4 \end{bmatrix}, C = \begin{bmatrix} C_1 & C_2 \\ C_3 & C_4 \end{bmatrix}, D = \begin{bmatrix} D_1 & D_2 \\ D_3 & D_4 \end{bmatrix}$. It can be easily found in the literature which additional properties do matrices A, B, C, D have to satisfy in order g_2 be an element of $SU(2,2)$. The result of the action of g_2 (or of just g, in terms of the Section 1 notation) on an element z from D = U(2) is as follows: $(Az + B)(Cz + D)^{-1}$.

Appendix B

(i.e., B1, B2, B3 - with a dent on top, or WD-case; B4 – no dent on top, or ND-case; the WD-, ND-terminology was introduced in our Section 5)

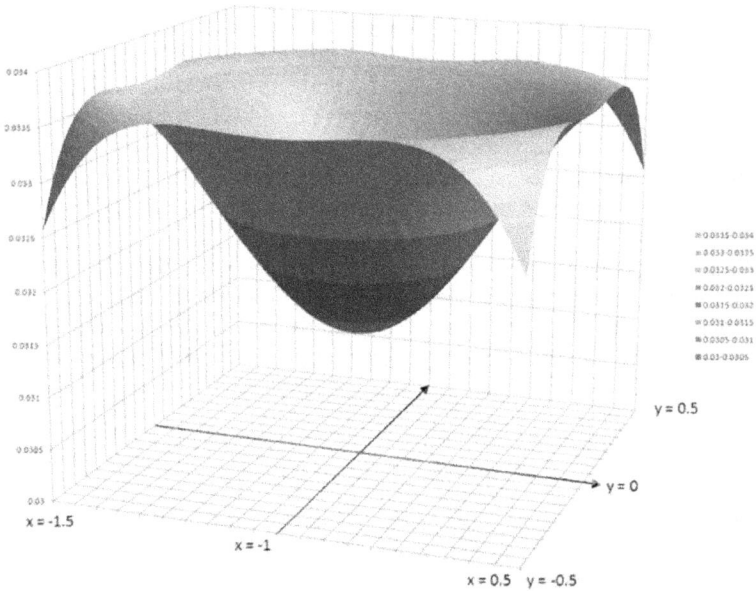

Figure B1.
An upper portion of the toy proton wave function.

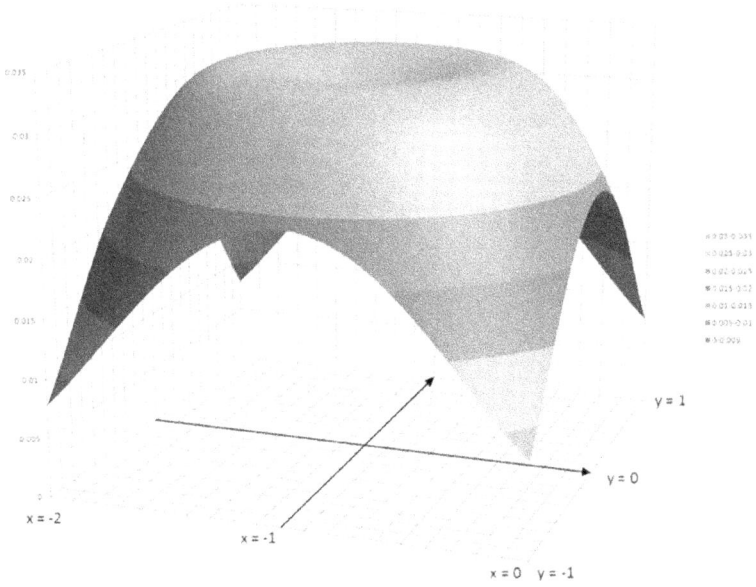

Figure B2.
A middle portion of the toy proton wave function.

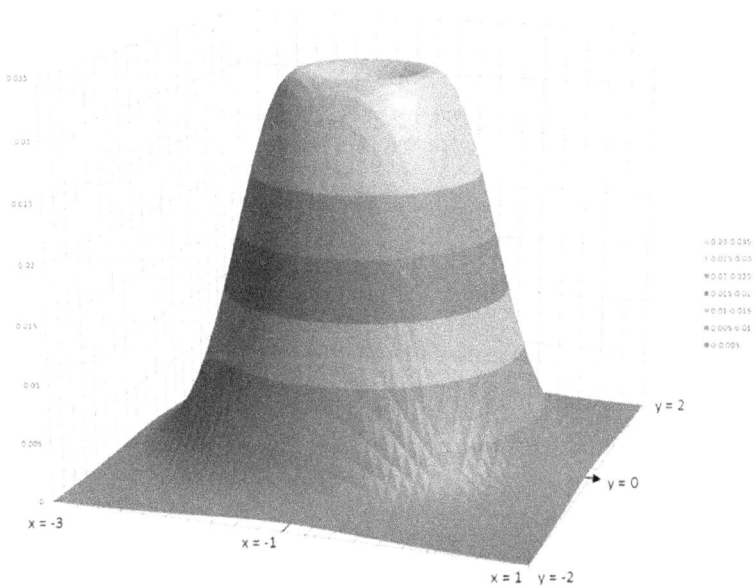

Figure B3.
The entire graph of the toy proton wave function.

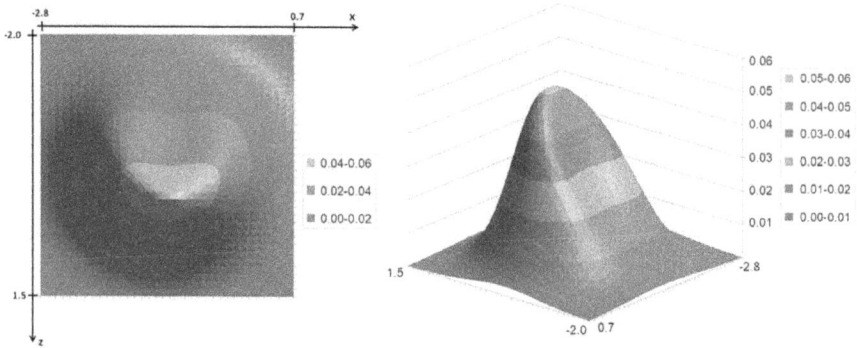

Figure B4.
On realistic 'sunken proton' wave function.

Author details

Yulia Klevtsova[1], Alexander Levichev[2*], Mikhail Neshchadim[3] and Andrey Palyanov[4]

1 Ershov Institute of Informatics Systems and Siberian State University of Telecommunications and Information Science, Novosibirsk, Russia

2 Sobolev Institute of Mathematics and Ershov Institute of Informatics Systems, Novosibirsk, Russia

3 Sobolev Institute of Mathematics, Novosibirsk, Russia

4 Ershov Institute of Informatics Systems and Novosibirsk State University, Novosibirsk, Russia

*Address all correspondence to: alevichev@gmail.com

IntechOpen

References

[1] Breidenbach M et al. Observed behavior of highly inelastic electron-proton scattering. Physical Review Letters. 1969;**23**:935-939

[2] Levichev AV. Towards a matrix multi-level model of quark-gluon media. JPRM [Internet]. 2016;**10**(2):1493-1496. Available from: http://scitecresearch.com/journals/index.php/jprm/article/view/974

[3] Levichev AV. One possible application of the chronometric theory of I.E. Segal: A toy model of quarks and gluons. Journal of Physics: Conference Series. 2019;**1194**:012071

[4] Segal IE. Is the cygnet the quintessential baryon? Proceedings of the National Academy of Sciences. 1991;**88**:994-998

[5] Wigner EP. On unitary representations of the inhomogeneous Lorentz group. Annals of Mathematics. 1939;**40**(2):149-204

[6] Levichev AV, Palyanov AY. On colors and electric charges of quarks: Modeling in terms of groups U(n) and SU(n,n). Mathematical Structures and Modeling. 2020;**4**(56):31-40, in Russian

[7] Levichev AV. On key properties of the intertwining operators ornament in the matrix multi-level model of the quark-gluon media. In: Proceedings of the All-Russia Conference with the International Participation "Knowledge-Ontology-Theories" (KONT-2017); 6–8 October 2017 Novosibirsk. Vol. 2. Novosibirsk: Sobolev Institute of Mathematics of the Siberian Division RAS; 2017. pp. 41-47

[8] Kon M, Levichev A. Parallelization analysis of space-time bundles and applications in particle physics. In: Proceedings of the All-Russia Conference with the International Participation "Knowledge-Ontology-Theories" (KONT-2019); 7–11 October 2019 Novosibirsk. Novosibirsk: Sobolev Institute of Mathematics of the Siberian Division RAS; 2019. pp. 385-392

[9] Levichev A, Palyanov A. Standard charges of quarks determination in terms of the multi-level model. In: Proceedings of the All-Russia Conference with the International Participation "Knowledge-Ontology-Theories" (KONT-2019); 7–11 October 2019 Novosibirsk. Novosibirsk: Sobolev Institute of Mathematics of the Siberian Division RAS; 2019. pp. 222-226

[10] Jakobsen HP, Levichev AV, Palyanov AY. The Wigner-Segal method as applied to the problem of quarks' and leptons' generations. In: Proceedings of the All-Russia Conference with the International Participation "Knowledge-Ontology-Theories" (KONT-2021); 8–12 November Novosibirsk. Novosibirsk: Sobolev Institute of Mathematics of the Siberian Division RAS; 2021. pp. 344-352. Available from: http://math.nsc.ru/conference/zont/21/index.htm

[11] Jakobsen HP, Levichev AV. The representation of SU(2,2) which is interpreted as describing chronometric fermions (proton, neutrino, and electron) in terms of a single composition series. Reports on Mathematical Physics. 2022;**90**(1):103-121

[12] Levichev A, Palyanov A. The multi-level model for quarks and leptons as the symbiosis of Segal's chronometry with the standard model. Preprint. 2022. 19 p. This version not peer-reviewed. Full publication to appear soon. DOI: 10.20944/preprints202202.0280.v1

[13] Levichev AV. Pseudo-hermitian realization of the Minkowski world through DLF theory. Physica Scripta. 2011;**83**:1-9. Available from: https://iopscience.iop.org/article/10.1088/0031-8949/83/01/015101

[14] Levichev AV. Segal's chronometry: Its development, application to the physics of particles and their interactions, further perspectives. In: Lavrent'ev M, Samoilov V, editors. Poisk matematicheskih zakonomernostei Mirozdania. Novosibirsk: GEO; 2010. pp. 66-99 in Russian

[15] Paneitz SM, Segal IE, Vogan DA Jr. Analysis in space-time bundles, IV. Journal of Functional Analysis. 1987;**75**:1-57

[16] Moylan P. Harmonic analysis on spannors. Journal of Mathematical Physics. 1995;**36**:2826-2879

[17] Jakobsen HP. Intertwining differential operators for Mp(n;R) and SU(n; n). Transactions of the American Mathematical Society. 1978;**246**:311-337

[18] Jakobsen HP, Vergne M. Wave and Dirac operators and representations of the conformal group. Journal of Functional Analysis. 1977;**24**:52-106

[19] Barut AOA. Return to 1932: Proton, electron and neutrino as true elementary constituents of leptons, hadrons and nuclei. In: Quantum Theory and the Structures of Time and Space. Vol. 4. Munich: Carl Hanser Press; 1981. pp. 152-163

[20] Varadarajan V. Geometry of Quantum Theory. New York: Springer; 1985. 412 p

[21] Faessler M. Weinberg angle and integer electric charges of quarks. arXiv. 2013. 6 p. Available from: https://arxiv.org/abs/1308.5900

[22] Levichev AV, Klevtsova Y, Palyanov A, Yu AD. Alexandrov would have been 110, and a contribution to chronometry. Mathematical Structures and Modeling. 2022;2(62):66-75 in Russian

[23] Qiu B, Men Y, Wang J, Hui Z. Dosimetry, efficacy, safety, and cost effectiveness of proton therapy for non-small cell lung cancer. Cancers (Basel). 2021;**13**(18):4545. DOI: 10.3390/cancers13184545. Available from: https://www.ncbi.nlm.nih.gov/pmc/articles/PMC8465697/

[24] Fitz, Gerald J, Bishop-Jodoin TM, editors. Dosimetry [Internet]. London, UK: IntechOpen; 2022. DOI: 10.5772/intechopen.98044

Chapter 3

Radiobiology of Proton Therapy and Its Clinical Implications

Eter Natelauri, Mariam Pkhaladze and Mikheil Atskvereli

Abstract

The chapter delves into the intricate relationship between proton therapy and its impact on biological systems, shaping the landscape of modern cancer treatment. Proton accelerators and beam delivery systems are discussed, followed by analyses of proton beam characterization, penumbra, and Bragg peak phenomena, and their impact on biological responses. Cellular responses to proton radiation encompass cell cycle dynamics, pathways to cell death, mitotic catastrophe, and senescence, oxygen enhancement ratios in hypoxic tumors, and modulation of inflammatory and immune responses. Radiobiological modeling emerges as a predictive tool. Linear-Quadratic models, biophysical models for radiosensitivity, clinical outcome modeling, and the advent of radiogenomics and personalized medicine shape treatment strategies. Pediatric patients demand specialized consideration. Unique aspects, late effects, clinical outcomes, and long-term follow-up, coupled with advancements in pediatric proton therapy, form the crux of this section. Spot-scanning and pencil beam scanning techniques, FLASH proton therapy, heavy ion therapy, and innovative approaches like radioprotectors and combining proton therapy with immunotherapy pave the way for the next era in cancer treatment. This chapter navigates the dynamic interplay of radiobiology, technology, and patient care, fostering a comprehensive understanding of proton therapy's potential in oncological practice.

Keywords: proton therapy, radiobiology, biological response, external beam, radiation therapy, radiation therapy biology, early and late adverse events

1. Introduction

Radiobiology encompasses a realm within clinical and fundamental medical sciences, focusing on the examination of how ionizing radiation impacts living organisms, particularly delving into the ramifications of radiation exposure on health. At the same time, radiotherapy has consistently upheld its status as a highly efficacious approach for treating cancer, finding its place in the management of approximately half of all patients at some stage of their care journey. Radiation treatment is commonly employed at various stages of cancer care, and it's often administered through photon-based intensity-modulated external beam therapy. However, technological advancements and research have enabled the development of charged particle therapies like intensity-modulated proton therapy. Proton beams have the unique property of depositing most of their energy at the end of their path, known as the Bragg peak.

This feature allows clinicians to deliver higher radiation doses to cancerous cells while sparing the surrounding healthy tissue. Unlike photon beams, which are low linear energy transfer (LET), proton beams, particularly those in the spread-out Bragg peak (SOBP), are high LET. This gives proton therapy not just a physical advantage in dose distribution, but also unique biological benefits compared to traditional photon radiation. While there is a wealth of research on how tumors and healthy tissues react to photon-based therapies, the biological responses to proton therapy are not yet fully understood. Without a doubt, radiobiology has proven to be highly productive in generating novel concepts and pinpointing potentially valuable mechanisms for treatment. This has resulted in the emergence of various innovative treatment approaches. Unfortunately, only a handful of these strategies have yielded evident clinical advantages thus far. However, the capacity of laboratory science to provide comprehensive guidance to radiotherapists for selecting precise protocols remains constrained by the insufficiency of theoretical and experimental models. Consequently, the ultimate selection of a protocol will invariably require reliance on outcomes from clinical trials.

2. Radiation interactions with matter

Radiation interactions with matter lie at the heart of understanding the intricate dance between particles and materials. This phenomenon forms the cornerstone of not only particle physics but also finds extensive application in medical imaging, radiation therapy, and diverse scientific fields (**Table 1**). Delving into the depths of these interactions provides crucial insights into the behavior of radiation as it traverses various substances, yielding valuable information that underpins both theoretical understanding and practical applications. The fundamental understanding of radiation-matter interactions is anchored in the profound concepts of ionization and excitation. Ionization involves the removal of electrons from atoms, resulting in charged species and the potential for subsequent chemical reactions. Excitation, on the other hand, involves the elevation of electrons to higher energy levels without

Photoelectric effect	In the photoelectric effect, an incident photon is absorbed by an atom, causing an inner-shell electron to be ejected. This mechanism is predominant at lower photon energies and is more probable in elements with higher atomic numbers (Z) [1].
Compton scattering	In Compton scattering, the incident photon is scattered by an electron, causing a change in the photon's direction and energy. The scattered photon has less energy, and the electron gains the energy difference [2].
Pair production	In pair production, a photon with energy greater than 1.02 MeV interacts near the nucleus and creates an electron-positron pair. The photon's energy is transformed into mass, following Einstein's $E = mc^2$ equation [3].
Coherent scattering	Also known as Rayleigh or classical scattering, coherent scattering involves the scattering of low-energy photons without any energy transfer [1].
Alpha particle interaction	Alpha particles have a + 2 charge and interact with matter through Coulomb forces. They have low penetration ability and can be stopped by a sheet of paper or skin [4].
Beta particle interaction	Beta particles are high-speed electrons or positrons. Their interaction with matter involves ionization and excitation of atoms along their path [5].

Table 1.
Mechanisms of interaction.

complete detachment. These processes unravel the intricacies of particle behavior as they lose energy to the surrounding matter [6].

The comprehension of these interactions has led to the development of medical imaging modalities that have revolutionized healthcare. In X-ray computed tomography (CT), the attenuation of X-rays as they pass through different tissues is harnessed to create detailed cross-sectional images. Understanding radiation interactions assists in optimizing CT protocols balancing image quality and patient dose. Similarly, positron emission tomography (PET) exploits the interaction between emitted positrons and electrons in the surrounding tissue, creating images that provide insights into metabolic processes at the molecular level [7]. Radiation therapy, a cornerstone of cancer treatment, harnesses the power of radiation-matter interactions to target and destroy cancer cells while minimizing damage to healthy tissues. Knowledge of these interactions aids in designing treatment plans that deliver precise doses to tumor sites based on tissue composition and density. Modern techniques like intensity-modulated radiation therapy (IMRT) and proton therapy rely on accurate predictions of radiation behavior in different tissues, optimizing treatment outcomes.

Ionizing radiation bestows its energy upon the medium it traverses, an interaction intrinsic to its path. The pivotal aspect of ionizing radiation's interaction with biological matter lies in the stochastic and discrete nature of energy deposition. Energy is distributed in progressively energetic packets referred to as "spurs" (when around 100 eV is deposited), "blobs" (for 100–500 eV), or "short tracks" (encompassing 500–5000 eV), with each packet leaving in its wake roughly three to several dozen ionized atoms. This depiction is visualized in **Figure 1**, accompanied by a proportionally scaled segment of (interphase) chromatin. The discrete nature of these energy deposition occurrences leads to a significant observation: while the average energy deposited within a macroscopic volume of biological material is modest, the distribution of this energy on a microscopic level can be substantial. This inherent characteristic contributes to ionizing radiation's exceptional effectiveness in generating biological damage. For instance, the energy deposited in a 70-kg human that results in a 50% probability of death amounts to approximately 70 calories, equivalent to the energy absorbed from a single sip of hot coffee. Notably, the distinction lies in the uniform distribution of energy in the coffee sip, as opposed to the random and discrete nature of ionizing radiation [8].

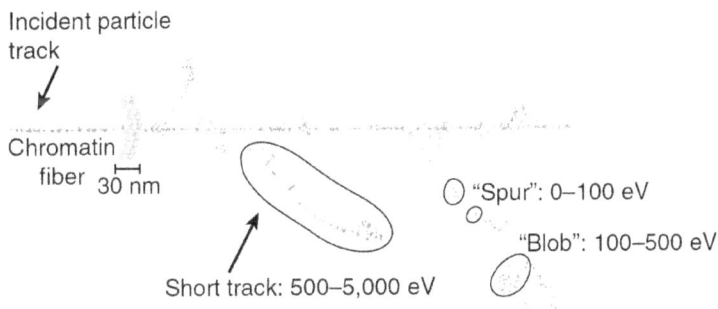

Figure 1.
Charged particle tracking through an absorbing medium, illustrating the random and discrete energy-deposition events along the track. Each event can be classified according to the amount of energy deposited locally, which determines how many ionized atoms will be produced. A segment of chromatin is shown approximately to scale.

Molecules directly struck by a spur or blob encounter a relatively elevated radiation dose, signifying substantial energy deposition within a confined volume. In the context of photons and charged particles, this energy deposition prompts the expulsion of orbital electrons from atoms, converting the target molecule initially into an ion pair and subsequently into a free radical [9]. Furthermore, the liberated electrons—themselves energetic charged particles—can instigate additional ionizations. Conversely, for uncharged particles like neutrons, interaction occurs between the incident particles and the nuclei of atoms within the absorbing medium. This interaction triggers the emission of recoil protons (charged particles) and lower-energy neutrons. This sequence of events, encompassing ionization, free radical generation, and release of secondary charged particles, persists until the entire energy of the incident photon or particle is dissipated. These interactions conclude within a mere picosecond following the initial energy transfer. Beyond this juncture, the ensuing chemical reactions of the resulting free radicals assume prominence, thus shaping the radiation response in subsequent time frames. The interaction of radiation with matter can produce various physical and chemical changes, which have both beneficial and harmful implications [4, 5].

Understanding radiation interactions with matter is vital for various applications like radiation therapy, radiography, and radiation shielding. Proper shielding materials and techniques can mitigate radiation exposure, depending on the type and energy of the radiation involved [10]. Understanding the mechanisms of how radiation interacts with matter is critical for harnessing its beneficial applications and mitigating its harmful effects. Each type of radiation interaction has specific characteristics, which must be accounted for in both technological applications and safety protocols.

Protons are ionized particles that can be propelled and directed into biological tissue to release their energy. The most prevalent form of heavy ion radiation treatment is proton therapy. What sets protons apart from conventional X-ray beams is their unique energy deposition profile: they provide a minimal radiation dose to the superficial, healthy tissues, peak at the depth where the tumor resides, and essentially offer no residual radiation to tissues beyond the tumor. This energy distribution is in stark contrast to that of x-rays, where the highest energy is generally absorbed by tissues closer to the surface. The Relative Biological Effectiveness (RBE) for protons stands at roughly 1.1, indicating only a slight biological advantage over x-rays or electrons (**Table 2**). The principal merit of proton therapy, therefore, lies in its optimized dose distribution [11].

The generation of proton beams involves the use of cyclotrons or synchrotrons to propel ionized hydrogen atoms to energy levels exceeding 160 Mega Electron Volts (MeV). The machinery required for this process is generally more expansive and costly compared to traditional linear accelerators, often requiring dedicated facilities. Protons behave differently from electrons in that they deposit their energy

X-ray	1
Gamma-rays	1
Beta particles	1
Protons	1.1–2
Alpha particles	20

Table 2.
The relative biological effectiveness for different types of radiation.

increasingly as they travel deeper into the tissue, leading to a concentrated area of dose deposition known as the Bragg peak. By adjusting the energy of the proton beams, the Bragg peak can be precisely positioned to maximize the dose at the tumor site, thereby minimizing exposure to healthy tissue. To ensure comprehensive treatment, a technique known as a Spread-Out Bragg Peak (SOBP) is employed, which involves adjusting the proton energy or using varying modulators to cover the entire target area with a uniform dose [12].

Clinical applications of proton therapy have primarily focused on prostate cancer, though empirical evidence proving its superiority in this context is still lacking. Proton therapy is especially advantageous for treating pediatric malignancies, particularly those of the central nervous system, due to its minimal impact on healthy tissues. Research on utilizing protons for treating lung cancer and other anatomical sites is underway. Given the substantial costs associated with proton therapy equipment and specialized facilities, there is an ongoing debate on whether the benefits justify the investment. Despite the lack of definitive evidence so far, the number of facilities offering proton therapy continues to grow even in developing countries.

Understanding radiation interactions with matter is indispensable in radiobiology, particularly in the context of proton therapy—an advanced form of radiotherapy that exploits the unique physical and biological properties of protons:

- Depth-dose distribution and penetration: unlike photons, protons have a mass and charge, leading to distinct depth-dose distributions. Proton beams can be modulated to deliver a more conformal dose to complex-shaped tumors, thanks to the unique control over the penetration depth afforded by manipulating the proton's initial kinetic energy [12].

- biological interactions: Linear Energy Transfer (LET) and Relative Biological effectiveness (RBE) [8].

  o Linear Energy Transfer (LET)—Protons exhibit a higher Linear Energy Transfer (LET) than photons, resulting in denser ionization tracks within the biological tissue. High-LET radiations are known to induce complex DNA damage, which is less amenable to repair mechanisms, thus enhancing the cytotoxic potential of the radiation.

  o Relative Biological Effectiveness (RBE)—The elevated LET of protons translates to a higher Relative Biological Effectiveness (RBE) compared to photons. RBE values are not constants but vary as a function of several variables including LET, dose, cell type, and even the phase of the cell cycle at the time of irradiation.

Normal tissues exhibit different levels of radiosensitivity based on cellular turnover, oxygenation status, and inherent DNA repair mechanisms. Cells in the G2 and M phases of the cell cycle are generally more radiosensitive than those in the G1 and S phases. Radiation can lead to various levels of cellular damage in normal tissues, ranging from sublethal damage repair to apoptosis and necrosis Organs like the skin, gut, and bone marrow are particularly sensitive due to their rapid cellular turnover. Tumors are often heterogeneous, comprising cells with varying degrees of radiosensitivity. Cancer stem cells within tumors may exhibit radioresistance, complicating eradication [13–16].

Tumor hypoxia is associated with increased radioresistance, largely due to the decreased availability of molecular oxygen that acts as a radiosensitizer. Many tumors have aberrant DNA repair mechanisms, which may either increase radiosensitivity due to impaired repair or promote radioresistance by more effective sublethal damage repair. Understanding the radiosensitivity of normal and tumor tissues allows for better planning and optimization of radiation therapy. New approaches like hypofractionation and targeted radionuclide therapy are being explored to maximize tumor cell kill while minimizing normal tissue damage [17–19]. Radiosensitivity varies significantly between normal tissues and tumor cells, with a multitude of factors contributing to these differences. Understanding these factors is critical for the effective use of radiation in medical applications and for mitigating the adverse effects of radiation exposure.

The cellular damage resulting from radiation primarily targets DNA, inducing single- or double-strand breaks. The efficiency of DNA repair mechanisms, including base excision repair and homologous recombination, varies between normal tissues and tumor cells, thereby contributing to their differential radiosensitivity. Apoptosis and Cell-Cycle Checkpoints—both normal and tumor cells have inherent mechanisms that determine their radiosensitivity, such as apoptosis and cell-cycle checkpoints. However, many tumor cells often have defects in these pathways, which may both enhance and compromise their radiosensitivity depending on the specific molecular context. The alpha-beta ratio (α/β ratio) is a metric widely used to quantify radiosensitivity, with a lower ratio generally indicating higher radiosensitivity. The α/β ratio for normal tissues often differs from that of tumor cells, a factor that must be considered in treatment planning [20]. The intrinsic radiosensitivity characteristics of tissues impact dose fractionation strategies in proton therapy. Sparing normal tissues while maximizing the dose to tumor cells is a primary goal that can be optimized by leveraging our understanding of radiosensitivity. In proton therapy, the higher RBE due to elevated LET can affect both tumor and normal tissue. Therefore, the differential radiosensitivity of normal and tumor tissues must be accurately incorporated into treatment planning algorithms. The advent of high throughput "omics" technologies and systems biology approaches are poised to bring new insights into the factors influencing radiosensitivity, which could lead to even more precise and personalized radiation therapy regimens.

3. Physical aspects of proton beam

Proton beam therapy relies on specialized accelerators to produce a high-energy beam of protons. The most commonly used accelerators for this purpose are cyclotrons and synchrotrons. A cyclotron uses a fixed magnetic field and variable electric field to accelerate protons in a spiral path, whereas a synchrotron uses a variable magnetic and electric field to accelerate protons in a circular path. Once the protons are accelerated to the desired energy level, they are delivered to the patient using a beam delivery system. The two primary methods for proton beam delivery are passive scattering and pencil beam scanning (PBS). In the passive scattering technique, the proton beam is broadened using a scatterer and then shaped using a collimator and compensator to conform to the target volume. In the PBS method, a narrow "pencil" beam of protons is scanned across the target volume, which allows for better dose conformity [21, 22].

Characterizing a proton beam involves several important parameters, including energy, fluence, and dose distribution. The energy of the beam determines its penetration depth in tissue. Proton beams are often characterized by their Bragg peak, where the dose deposition is maximized. The fluence of the beam indicates the number of protons per unit area and plays a role in the overall dose delivered to the tissue [23]. Additionally, imaging techniques like Positron Emission Tomography (PET) can be employed for in-vivo dose verification, thus adding another layer of safety and precision [24].

A unique characteristic of proton beams is the Bragg peak, a region where the energy deposition reaches a maximum, allowing for the precise targeting of cancer cells while sparing surrounding healthy tissue [21]. The "penumbra" refers to the region around the target volume where the dose falls off rapidly. In conventional X-ray therapy, the penumbra is relatively large, which can result in a higher dose to surrounding tissues. However, in proton therapy, the penumbra can be much smaller, allowing for a more targeted treatment [25].

The physical properties of the proton beam have a direct impact on its biological efficacy. Due to the Bragg peak, proton beams can deliver a higher dose to the target tissue while minimizing the dose to surrounding tissues. However, it's also important to note that high-linear energy transfer (LET) radiation like proton beams can produce complex DNA damage, which may result in different biological responses compared to low-LET radiation like X-rays. Moreover, proton therapy allows for hypofractionation, delivering higher doses per fraction, thus potentially reducing the overall treatment time [26, 27]. Research is ongoing to understand the biological consequences of varying beam properties, including energy, fluence, and dose rate, and their impact on the therapeutic ratio.

4. Proton-induced DNA damage

Understanding proton-induced DNA damage is essential for assessing the biological effectiveness and safety of proton therapy. This section elucidates various forms of DNA damage induced by protons, the repair mechanisms involved, and the biological significance of such damage. One of the most significant types of DNA damage caused by proton radiation is the double-strand break (DSB). DSBs occur when both strands of the DNA helix are severed, which could lead to chromosomal aberrations if not accurately repaired. Proton beams, owing to their high linear energy transfer (LET), are effective in inducing DSBs, which could make them more effective in killing cancer cells (**Figure 2**). Unlike conventional X-rays, high-LET radiation like

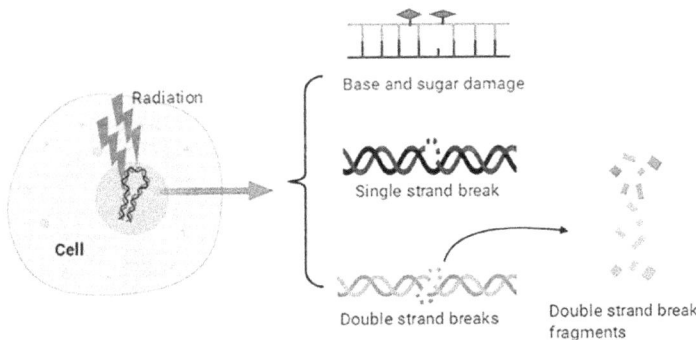

Figure 2.
DNA image induced by ionizing radiation. The major types of DNA damage induced by IR include base and sugar damage, single-strand breaks, double-strand breaks, clustered DNA damage, and covalent intrastrand or interstrand crosslinking.

protons can cause clustered DNA damage, where multiple types of lesions occur in proximity. This makes the repair process more complicated and increases the likelihood of misrepair and mutagenesis. Clustered DNA damage could include a combination of single-strand breaks, double-strand breaks, and base lesions, which collectively present a considerable challenge to cellular repair machinery [28–31].

The cellular machinery employs various mechanisms to repair DNA damage caused by proton radiation. These mechanisms include Non-Homologous End Joining (NHEJ) and Homologous Recombination (HR) for repairing double-strand breaks. For clustered DNA damage, specialized proteins like Rad52 and the MRN complex are involved in recognizing and flagging these complex lesions for repair. However, it's essential to note that the efficiency of these repair mechanisms can vary depending on various factors, such as the cell cycle phase and the presence of oxygen, which can modulate the effectiveness of proton therapy [32–34].

The biological implications of proton-induced DNA damage are multi-faceted. On the one hand, the effectiveness of proton beams in causing double-strand breaks and clustered damage makes it a potent therapeutic modality for cancer treatment. However, the complexity of proton-induced damage also raises concerns about the long-term effects, such as secondary cancers and normal tissue complications. Understanding these biological outcomes is crucial for optimizing proton therapy parameters, like dose and fractionation, to maximize therapeutic gain while minimizing collateral damage to normal tissues [29, 35, 36].

5. Cellular and molecular responses to proton radiation

Understanding the complex cellular and molecular responses to proton radiation is key to unlocking the full therapeutic potential of this modality. This section will delve into various pathways and mechanisms activated in response to proton radiation, including cell cycle arrest, cell death pathways, and the involvement of hypoxic conditions and immune responses. Exposure to proton radiation can trigger a series of cellular events leading to cell cycle arrest, primarily at the G1/S and G2/M checkpoints. This halt in the cell cycle allows cells to repair damaged DNA before proceeding to cell division, thus minimizing the risk of mutations and genomic instability. Several cell death pathways may be activated by proton radiation, including apoptosis, necrosis, and autophagy. The choice between these pathways is influenced by several factors, such as the extent of DNA damage, cellular context, and the activation of specific signaling pathways like p53 [37–40].

In cases where cell cycle checkpoints are bypassed or malfunctioning, cells may enter a state known as mitotic catastrophe. This is an onco-suppressive mechanism leading to the death of cells that have undergone aberrant mitosis [41]. Senescence is another cellular fate in response to proton irradiation. It leads to a state of irreversible growth arrest but not to cell death. The senescent cells, however, secrete pro-inflammatory cytokines, which can have a complex influence on the tumor microenvironment [42]. The presence of oxygen can significantly impact the efficacy of radiation therapies, including proton therapy. The oxygen enhancement ratio (OER) is a measure of how much more effective radiation is in the presence of oxygen compared to hypoxic conditions. Proton beams have been suggested to have a lower OER compared to X-rays, making them potentially more effective in treating hypoxic tumors [43].

Proton radiation can modulate the tumor microenvironment, particularly affecting the inflammatory and immune responses. For instance, protons can stimulate the release of cytokines such as IL-6 and TNF-α, which play roles in both promoting and suppressing tumor growth [44]. Furthermore, proton radiation has been shown to increase the presentation of tumor antigens, thereby enhancing the anti-tumor immune response [45]. Understanding these complex interactions can guide the optimization of proton therapy regimens and may pave the way for combination treatments involving immunotherapies.

6. Radiobiological models and treatment outcome prediction

The translation of proton therapy from a conceptual tool to a clinically effective treatment requires an integration of radiobiological knowledge with technological advances. Radiobiological models serve as invaluable instruments in predicting treatment outcomes, identifying the best treatment regimens, and offering personalized therapeutic approaches. This section elaborates on various models and their significance in optimizing proton therapy.

The Linear-Quadratic (LQ) model is commonly used to describe the dose-response relationship for cell survival after radiation exposure. Originally developed for photon radiation, the LQ model has been adapted to fit the complex biological responses to proton therapy [46]. The model estimates cell survival by considering both linear and quadratic terms of radiation dose, with alpha and beta as tissue-specific constants. In proton therapy, the LQ model can be adjusted to account for the variations in Linear Energy Transfer (LET) along the Bragg peak, thus providing a more accurate description of the dose-response relationship [47]. Apart from the LQ model, there are biophysical models like the Microdosimetric Kinetic Model (MKM) and the Local Effect Model (LEM), which aim to predict cellular radiosensitivity. These models consider the geometric and molecular complexities of cellular structures, thereby offering a more nuanced understanding of proton-induced biological effects [48, 49]. Such models are particularly useful in the treatment planning stage to optimize the dose distribution based on the predicted radiosensitivity of both tumor and normal tissues.

Beyond theoretical predictions, radiobiological models have been increasingly incorporated into clinical research to predict outcomes for specific cancers treated with proton therapy. By integrating various clinical, dosimetric, and biological factors, these models can estimate treatment efficacy, survival rates, and the risk of complications [50]. For instance, models that incorporate tumor volume, prescribed dose, and patient age have been developed to predict the probability of tumor control and normal tissue toxicity in treatments like head and neck or prostate cancers [51].

With the advent of high-throughput genomic technologies, the field of radiogenomics has emerged to identify genetic markers that could predict individual responses to radiation. Integrating radiogenomic data into radiobiological models opens the door to personalized proton therapy, where treatment plans are tailored to the individual's unique genetic and molecular profile. By leveraging machine learning algorithms and big data analytics, researchers are making strides in identifying robust radiogenomic markers that could be implemented in routine clinical practice [52–54].

7. Adverse effects and normal tissue toxicity

One of the significant challenges in radiation therapy, including proton therapy, is striking a balance between maximizing tumor control and minimizing normal tissue toxicity. Understanding the early and late effects of proton radiation on normal tissues is paramount for optimizing treatment plans and improving patient outcomes. This section will explore the different types of radiation-induced effects and how normal tissue tolerances are considered in proton therapy.

7.1 Radiation-induced early effects

Proton therapy has been gaining traction as a preferred modality for cancer treatment due to its ability to deliver highly conformal doses of radiation to the target while sparing surrounding normal tissues [55, 56]. However, like any other form of radiation therapy, proton therapy is not devoid of side effects. It is crucial to understand the early adverse effects induced by proton therapy to establish safe and efficient treatment protocols. This section aims to elucidate the early adverse effects of proton radiation therapy, offering a comprehensive review of the underlying mechanisms, clinical manifestations, and mitigation strategies.

Radiation-induced early effects are typically observed during or shortly after the course of treatment and may include skin erythema, mucositis, and acute gastrointestinal symptoms. These effects are usually reversible but can have an impact on the patient's quality of life and compliance with the treatment regimen. The nature and severity of early effects can vary depending on the tissue type, dose per fraction, and total dose, among other factors [57–59].

One of the key factors contributing to early adverse effects in proton therapy is the interaction of proton beams with biological tissues. Unlike traditional photon beams, proton beams have high linear energy transfer (LET), especially at the Bragg peak, where most of the energy is deposited [60]. High LET radiation is more efficient at ionizing biological molecules, increasing the risk of early tissue reactions including inflammation and skin erythema [61].

Gastrointestinal (GI) toxicity is a common early side effect observed in patients undergoing proton therapy for abdominal and pelvic malignancies [62]. Symptoms may include nausea, vomiting, and diarrhea. Early GI toxicity is believed to result from the radiation-induced apoptosis of the rapidly dividing epithelial cells lining the GI tract [63]. Radiation dermatitis is another frequently reported early adverse effect of proton therapy [64]. This usually presents as redness, itching, or even skin ulceration at the site of radiation. The likelihood of developing dermatitis is dependent on various factors such as dose, fractionation, and individual patient sensitivity [65]. In instances where radiation fields include bone marrow, patients may experience early hematological changes including leucopenia and thrombocytopenia [66]. These conditions can lead to increased susceptibility to infections and may require dose modifications or delays in treatment [67].

Efforts to mitigate these early adverse effects include modifying treatment plans, optimizing dose distribution, and incorporating pharmaceutical interventions such as anti-inflammatory medications or antihistamines [68, 69]. Additionally, advancements in proton therapy technology, such as pencil-beam scanning, hold promise for minimizing these early adverse effects by allowing more precise dose distributions [70].

Understanding the early adverse effects of proton therapy is pivotal for clinicians to make informed decisions about treatment protocols. While proton therapy offers several advantages over traditional photon-based treatments, early adverse effects such as GI toxicity, dermatitis, and hematological changes remain areas of concern that necessitate ongoing research and clinical attention.

7.2 Radiation-induced late effects

In contrast to early effects, radiation-induced late effects may manifest several months or years post-treatment and can have a more severe impact on the patient's long-term well-being. These can include fibrosis, cognitive impairment, and secondary cancers. Late effects are particularly concerning because they are often irreversible and can progressively worsen over time. Research has shown that proton therapy may offer a lower incidence of late effects compared to conventional photon therapy, primarily because of its precision and reduced scatter [71–73].

Late cardiopulmonary complications can manifest as myocardial fibrosis, coronary artery disease, or even lung fibrosis [74]. Studies suggest that these effects might be attributed to the scattering of protons in tissues with high atomic numbers, such as bones surrounding the chest cavity [75]. Patients treated with proton therapy for brain tumors may face delayed neurological effects, including cognitive decline and neuroendocrine dysfunction [76]. These adverse effects are thought to stem from the high linear energy transfer (LET) properties of protons causing greater damage to sensitive neural structures [77]. One of the most concerning late effects is the increased risk of secondary malignancies. Unlike photon radiation, which dissipates energy throughout the treatment volume, protons deposit the majority of their energy at the Bragg peak. However, the entrance dose and neutron scatter can still induce DNA mutations that may lead to secondary cancers [78]. Late effects can also impact the musculoskeletal system, causing fibrosis or even necrosis of the bone and surrounding tissues [79]. These are particularly of concern in pediatric populations, where proton therapy is commonly used to treat bone tumors [80]. Late gastrointestinal complications like strictures or fistulas can occur post-treatment for abdominal and pelvic cancers. These are thought to result from the delayed effects of radiation on the vascular supply and fibroblast proliferation in the gut lining [81].

Several strategies have been proposed for the management and mitigation of late adverse effects. Dose-volume histograms and biological effective dose (BED) calculations are used to predict the risk of late toxicity. Hypofractionation and integration of radioprotective drugs are being investigated as potential strategies to minimize the incidence of late effects [62, 82]. While proton therapy offers a sophisticated and precise approach to cancer treatment, clinicians must remain vigilant for potential late adverse effects. Ongoing research aims to further understand these complications and develop effective strategies for their prevention and management.

7.3 Normal tissue tolerance in proton therapy

Normal tissue tolerance is a critical parameter in treatment planning. Radiation oncologists must understand the dose-volume constraints for various organs at risk (OARs) to minimize normal tissue toxicity. In proton therapy, the normal tissue complication probability (NTCP) models are frequently employed to predict the likelihood of adverse effects in normal tissues. Given the distinct dosimetric profile of proton beams, especially the sharp dose fall-off beyond the Bragg peak, treatment planning in proton therapy often allows for better sparing of normal tissues. However, it is essential to continuously update and refine these models based on accumulating clinical evidence to ensure their applicability and accuracy in proton therapy settings [21, 83, 84].

8. Proton therapy and pediatric patients

Pediatric patients present a unique challenge in the context of radiation oncology, with considerations that are markedly different from adult populations. Proton therapy, known for its precision and reduced off-target effects, has been increasingly adopted for the treatment of pediatric malignancies. This section explores the unique considerations for pediatric patients undergoing proton therapy, the long-term effects of the treatment, clinical outcomes, and advancements in the field. Pediatric patients have a higher sensitivity to radiation, largely due to their developing tissues and organs. They are also at greater risk for secondary malignancies later in life following radiation exposure [85]. Proton therapy can be especially beneficial for this demographic because its precise targeting minimizes exposure to surrounding tissues, thereby reducing both immediate and long-term side effects [86]. Another challenge in pediatric proton therapy is the issue of growth and development. Treatment plans need to be adaptable to the physiological changes that occur as the child grows. This often requires more frequent adjustments to treatment plans compared to adults.

The late effects of proton therapy on pediatric patients can be profound, given their longer life expectancy post-treatment. Late effects may include growth abnormalities, neurocognitive deficits, and hormonal imbalances [73]. However, proton therapy's precision often results in fewer such effects compared to traditional photon radiation [87]. Understanding the long-term consequences requires extensive follow-up studies to inform future clinical practice. Therefore, a multi-disciplinary approach involving oncologists, endocrinologists, and neurologists is often necessary for monitoring and managing late effects in pediatric patients.

The long-term follow-up of pediatric patients treated with proton therapy shows promising outcomes. For various pediatric cancers, including medulloblastoma and rhabdomyosarcoma, proton therapy has demonstrated comparable or superior survival rates with reduced toxicity compared to photon therapy [88]. Long-term studies also show lower rates of secondary malignancies [89]. However, long-term follow-up is critical, given the vulnerability of this population to late effects. Regular assessments are essential for the early detection of any secondary malignancies or other complications.

9. Advanced techniques and combinatorial approaches in proton therapy

Advancements in radiation oncology have led to new and refined methods in proton therapy. This section explores some of these cutting-edge approaches, including advanced scanning techniques, FLASH proton therapy, heavy ion therapy, and the integration of proton therapy with pharmacological agents and immunotherapy. Spot-scanning and pencil beam scanning are two advanced techniques that offer enhanced dose conformity in proton therapy. These approaches are particularly useful for treating tumors with complex shapes and those located near critical structures [47]. Spot-scanning employs individual spots of radiation that are distributed layer by layer to construct a three-dimensional dose distribution [90]. Pencil beam scanning is a more advanced version, using a narrow proton beam that can be modulated in intensity.

These techniques offer higher flexibility in shaping the dose distribution, thereby reducing the dose to surrounding normal tissue and increasing the dose to the target volume.

FLASH proton therapy is an innovative approach delivering extremely high dose rates within ultra-short periods. Preliminary studies suggest that FLASH therapy might offer a greater therapeutic index by reducing toxicity to normal tissues while maintaining or enhancing the tumor-killing effect [91, 92]. The exact mechanisms behind these phenomena are still under investigation. Heavy ion therapy, such as carbon ion therapy, provides another option for increasing the biological effectiveness of radiation. Carbon ions offer a higher linear energy transfer (LET) compared to protons, making them potentially more effective for hypoxic or radioresistant tumors [93]. Ongoing research aims to determine the optimal use cases for heavy ion therapy and its comparative effectiveness against proton therapy [94].

Pharmacological agents such as radioprotectors can be employed to minimize toxicity to normal tissues, while radiosensitizers can enhance the tumor-killing effect of radiation [95]. When used in combination with proton therapy, these agents may offer new ways to improve the therapeutic ratio. However, the use of these agents needs to be carefully considered due to their potential interactions and side effects.

There is growing interest in combining proton therapy with immunotherapeutic agents to exploit potential synergies in cancer treatment. Proton therapy may induce immunogenic cell death, which can be further augmented by checkpoint inhibitors and other immunotherapeutic strategies. Clinical trials are underway to evaluate the effectiveness of this combinatorial approach [96, 97].

10. Conclusion

The realm of proton radiobiology has evolved substantially over the years, demonstrating a complex interplay of physical, biological, and clinical factors that culminate in therapeutic outcomes. From its inception, proton therapy has been heralded as a significant step forward in radiation oncology, with its key feature being the ability to deliver highly conformal radiation doses to tumors while sparing adjacent healthy tissues. Nevertheless, while the physical aspects of proton therapy have been relatively well understood, it's only in recent years that the biological underpinnings have begun to be elucidated in greater detail.

The interaction of protons with biological tissues, particularly at the cellular and sub-cellular levels, offers both opportunities and challenges. The advantageous dose distributions characterized by the Bragg peak provide the theoretical underpinning for the utility of proton therapy. However, biological factors such as variable radiosensitivity across cell types, DNA repair mechanisms, and the influence of the tumor microenvironment add layers of complexity that require a multidisciplinary approach to unravel. The use of proton therapy in special populations, such as pediatric patients, has drawn significant attention. Here, the reduction of late effects and secondary malignancies becomes particularly crucial, and proton therapy holds the promise of more favorable outcomes. However, these benefits need to be systematically validated through long-term follow-up studies, incorporating advances in treatment planning and delivery.

Advancements in treatment techniques, such as spot-scanning, pencil beam scanning, and FLASH proton therapy, offer new avenues to improve dose delivery and possibly therapeutic outcomes. Moreover, combinatorial approaches incorporating heavy ion therapy, radioprotectors, radiosensitizers, and immunotherapy provide exciting prospects for enhancing the effectiveness of proton therapy. These advancements are particularly critical when considering the varied response of different tumor types and anatomical locations to proton therapy.

Despite these developments, several challenges remain. The limited availability of proton therapy centers, the high costs associated with the technology, and the need for more definitive comparative studies to validate its superiority over traditional therapies are all hurdles that the field must overcome. Furthermore, as more becomes known about the biological mechanisms underpinning the interactions between protons and tissues, there will be a growing need for models that can integrate these diverse sets of data into predictive frameworks for patient outcomes.

In conclusion, the field of proton radiobiology is a dynamic and evolving discipline that holds great promise for improving cancer treatment. As we continue to accumulate more data and refine our understanding of both the physical and biological aspects of this modality, it is crucial that we also focus on translating these findings into clinical practice. This will require a concerted effort from physicists, biologists, clinicians, and policymakers alike to ensure that the full therapeutic potential of proton therapy is realized.

Acknowledgements

We want to thank the people working at JCS VIAN and Krystyna Kiel Oncology Center for their encouragement and advice that led to the completion of this paper.

We also thank our friends and colleagues for their encouragement and words of advice.

Special thanks to our mentor—Krystyna Kiel, MD.

Finally, if not for our families, who supports us all the time, we would never be able to work on this extraordinary project.

Conflict of interest

The authors declared no potential conflicts of interest concerning the research, authorship, and/or publication of this article. This research did not receive a specific grant from funding agencies in the public, commercial, or not-for-profit sectors.

Author details

Eter Natelauri*, Mariam Pkhaladze and Mikheil Atskvereli
VIAN—Krystyna Kiel Oncology Center, Kutaisi, Georgia

*Address all correspondence to: enatelauri@vian.health

IntechOpen

References

[1] Podgorsak EB, Hendee WR. Radiation physics for medical physicists. Medical Physics. 2005;**33**(1):249

[2] Turner JE. Atoms, radiation and radiation protection 3 comp rev and enl ed. Weinheim, Germany: Wiley-VCH; 2007. 607 p. ISBN 978-3-527-40606-7. Worldcat

[3] Krane KS, Halliday D. Introductory Nuclear Physics. Kanada: John Wiley & Sons. Inc.; 1988

[4] Knoll GF. Radiation Detection and Measurement. 4th Edition. Hoboken, Germany: John Wiley & Sons; 2010. pp. 217. ISBN: 0470131489, 9780470131480

[5] Attix FH. Introduction to Radiological Physics and Radiation Dosimetry. Germany: John Wiley & Sons; 2008. ISBN: 978-3-527-61714-2

[6] Joiner MC, van der Kogel AJ, editors. Basic Clinical Radiobiology. 5th ed. Boca Raton: CRC Press; 2018. DOI: 10.1201/9780429490606. eBook. ISBN: 9780429490606

[7] Hall EJ, Giaccia AJ. Technologies Inc. Radiobiology for the Radiologist. 7th ed. Philadelphia: Wolters Kluwer Health and Lippincott Williams & Wilkins; 2012. Available from: http://ovidsp.ovid.com/ovidweb.cgi?T=JS&PAGE=booktext&NEWS=N&DF=bookdb&AN=01438882/7th_Edition&XPATH=/PG(0)

[8] Zeman EM. Biologic basis of radiation oncology. In: Gunderson LL, Tepper JS, editors. Clinical Radiation Oncology. 4th ed. Philadelphia: Elsevier; 2016

[9] Mettler FA, Upton AC. Medical Effects of Ionizing Radiation. 3rd ed. AJNR: American Journal of Neuroradiology. Philadelphia: Saunders Elsevier; 2009;**30**(2):e30. DOI: 10.3174/ajnr.A1289. PMCID: PMC7051411

[10] Martin A. Radiation Protection: A Guide for Scientists, Regulators, and Physicians. London, UK: Harvard University Press; 2006. ISBN: 9780674007406

[11] Tseng YD, Halasz L. Description of proton therapy. In: Principles of Neurological Surgery. Philadelphia, PA: Elsevier; 2018. pp. 736-744. ISBN: 978-0-323-43140-8

[12] Mohan R. Principles of proton beam therapy. In: Proton Therapy: Indications, Techniques and Outcomes. Philadelphia, Pennsylvania: Elsevier; 2020. p. 14-24. DOI: 10.1016/B978-0-323-73349-6.00011-X

[13] Pacelli R, Mansi L, Hall E, Giaccia AJ. Radiobiology for the radiologist. European Journal of Nuclear Medicine and Molecular Imaging. 6th ed. Philadelphia, USA: Lippincott Wilkins & Williams; 2006;**34**:965-966. DOI: 10.1007/s00259-007-0383-8. ISBN: 0-7817-4151-3

[14] Harrington L, Bristow RG, Hill RP, Tannock IF. Introduction to cancer biology. The Basic Science of Oncology. 2005;**4**:1-3

[15] Bristow RG, Hill RP. Hypoxia, DNA repair and genetic instability. Nature Reviews Cancer. 2008;**8**(3):180-192. DOI: 10.1038/nrc2344

[16] Diehn M, Cho RW, Lobo NA, Kalisky T, Dorie MJ, Kulp AN, et al. Association of reactive oxygen species levels and radioresistance in cancer stem cells. Nature. 2009;**458**(7239):780-783

[17] Brown JM, Wilson WR. Exploiting tumour hypoxia in cancer treatment. Nature Reviews Cancer. 2004;**4**(6):437-447

[18] Helleday T, Petermann E, Lundin C, Hodgson B, Sharma RA. DNA repair pathways as targets for cancer therapy. Nature Reviews Cancer. 2008;**8**(3):193-204

[19] Baumann M, Krause M, Overgaard J, Debus J, Bentzen SM, Daartz J, et al. Radiation oncology in the era of precision medicine. Nature Reviews Cancer. 2016;**16**(4):234-249

[20] Van Leeuwen CM, Oei AL, Crezee J, Bel A, Franken NA, Stalpers LJ, et al. The alfa and beta of tumours: A review of parameters of the linear-quadratic model, derived from clinical radiotherapy studies. Radiation Oncology. 2018;**13**(1):1-1

[21] Paganetti H, Gottschalk B, Schippers M, Lu HM, Flanz J, Slopsema R, editors. Proton Therapy Physics. 2nd ed. Boca Raton: CRC Press; 2018. DOI: 10.1201/b22053. ISBN: 9781315228310

[22] Schippers JM, Lomax AJ. Emerging technologies in proton therapy. Acta Oncologica. 2011;**50**(6):838-850

[23] Newhauser WD, Zhang R. The physics of proton therapy. Physics in Medicine & Biology. 2015;**60**(8):R155

[24] Parodi K, Polf JC. In vivo range verification in particle therapy. Medical Physics. 2018;**45**(11):e1036-e1050

[25] Darafsheh A, editor. Radiation Therapy Dosimetry: A Practical Handbook. 1st ed. Boca Raton: CRC Press; 2021. DOI: 10.1201/9781351005388. eBook. ISBN: 9781351005388

[26] Girdhani S, Sachs R, Hlatky L. Biological effects of proton radiation: What we know and don't know. Radiation Research. 2013;**179**(3):257-272

[27] Kirkby C, Mackay RI. An introduction to proton therapy physics. Physics in Medicine & Biology. 2013;**58**(11):R221

[28] Löbrich M, Jeggo PA. The impact of a negligent G2/M checkpoint on genomic instability and cancer induction. Nature Reviews Cancer. 2007;**7**(11):861-869

[29] Sørensen BS, Bassler N, Nielsen S, Horsman MR, Grzanka L, Spejlborg H, et al. Relative biological effectiveness (RBE) and distal edge effects of proton radiation on early damage in vivo. Acta Oncologica. 2017;**56**(11):1387-1391

[30] Sage E, Shikazono N. Radiation-induced clustered DNA lesions: Repair and mutagenesis. Free Radical Biology and Medicine. 2017;**107**:125-135

[31] Goodhead DT. Initial events in the cellular effects of ionizing radiations: Clustered damage in DNA. International Journal of Radiation Biology. 1994;**65**(1):7-17

[32] Chapman JR, Taylor MR, Boulton SJ. Playing the end game: DNA double-strand break repair pathway choice. Molecular Cell. 2012;**47**(4):497-510

[33] Stenerlöw B, Karlsson KH, Cooper B, Rydberg B. Measurement of prompt DNA double-strand breaks in mammalian cells without including heat-labile sites: Results for cells deficient in nonhomologous end joining. Radiation Research. 2003;**159**(4):502-510

[34] Chaudhary P, Marshall TI, Perozziello FM, Manti L, Currell FJ, Hanton F, et al. Relative biological

effectiveness variation along monoenergetic and modulated Bragg peaks of a 62-MeV therapeutic proton beam: A preclinical assessment. International Journal of Radiation Oncology, Biology and Physics. 2014;**90**(1):27-35

[35] Friedland W, Schmitt E, Kundrát P, Dingfelder M, Baiocco G, Barbieri S, et al. Comprehensive track-structure based evaluation of DNA damage by light ions from radiotherapy-relevant energies down to stopping. Scientific Reports. 2017;**7**(1):45161

[36] Newhauser WD, Durante M. Assessing the risk of second malignancies after modern radiotherapy. Nature Reviews Cancer. 2011;**11**(6):438-448

[37] Bartek J, Lukas J. Mammalian G1-and S-phase checkpoints in response to DNA damage. Current Opinion in Cell Biology. 2001;**13**(6):738-747

[38] Sancar A, Lindsey-Boltz LA, Ünsal-Kaçmaz K, Linn S. Molecular mechanisms of mammalian DNA repair and the DNA damage checkpoints. Annual Review of Biochemistry. 2004;**73**(1):39-85

[39] Galluzzi L, Vitale I, Abrams JM, Alnemri ES, Baehrecke EH, Blagosklonny MV, et al. Molecular definitions of cell death subroutines: Recommendations of the nomenclature committee on cell death 2012. Cell Death & Differentiation. 2012;**19**(1):107-120

[40] Haupt S, Berger M, Goldberg Z, Haupt Y. Apoptosis-the p53 network. Journal of Cell Science. 2003;**116**(20):4077-4085

[41] Klein K, He K, Younes AI, Barsoumian HB, Chen D, Ozgen T, et al. Role of mitochondria in cancer immune evasion and potential therapeutic approaches. Frontiers in immunology. 2020;**11**:2622

[42] Campisi J. Aging, cellular senescence, and cancer. Annual Review of Physiology. 2013;**75**:685-705

[43] Wenzl T, Wilkens JJ. Modelling of the oxygen enhancement ratio for ion beam radiation therapy. Physics in Medicine & Biology. 2011;**56**(11):3251

[44] Deng L, Liang H, Xu M, Yang X, Burnette B, Arina A, et al. STING-dependent cytosolic DNA sensing promotes radiation-induced type I interferon-dependent antitumor immunity in immunogenic tumors. Immunity. 2014;**41**(5):843-852

[45] Durante M, Formenti SC. Radiation-induced chromosomal aberrations and immunotherapy: Micronuclei, cytosolic DNA, and interferon-production pathway. Frontiers in Oncology. 2018;**8**:192

[46] Fowler JF. The linear-quadratic formula and progress in fractionated radiotherapy. The British Journal of Radiology. 1989;**62**(740):679-694

[47] Paganetti H. Relative biological effectiveness (RBE) values for proton beam therapy. Variations as a function of biological endpoint, dose, and linear energy transfer. Physics in Medicine & Biology. 2014;**59**(22):R419

[48] Hawkins RB. A statistical theory of cell killing by radiation of varying linear energy transfer. Radiation Research. 1994;**140**(3):366-374

[49] Elsässer T, Scholz M. Cluster effects within the local effect model. Radiation Research. 2007;**167**(3):319-329

[50] Cheng Q, Roelofs E, Ramaekers BL, Eekers D, van Soest J, Lustberg T, et al.

Development and evaluation of an online three-level proton vs photon decision support prototype for head and neck cancer–comparison of dose, toxicity and cost-effectiveness. Radiotherapy and Oncology. 2016;**118**(2):281-285

[51] Fontanilla HP, Klopp AH, Lindberg ME, Jhingran A, Kelly P, Takiar V, et al. Anatomic distribution of [18F] fluorodeoxyglucose-avid lymph nodes in patients with cervical cancer. Practical Radiation Oncology. 2013;**3**(1):45-53

[52] West C, Rosenstein BS. Establishment of a radiogenomics consortium. International Journal of Radiation Oncology, Biology, Physics. 2010;**76**(5):1295-1296

[53] Kerns SL, West L, et al. Radiogenomics: The search for genetic predictors of radiotherapy response. Future Oncology. 2014;**10**(15):2391-2406

[54] Scott JG, Berglund A, Schell MJ, Mihaylov I, Fulp WJ, Yue B, et al. A genome-based model for adjusting radiotherapy dose (GARD): A retrospective, cohort-based study. The Lancet Oncology. 2017;**18**(2):202-211

[55] Mohan R. A review of proton therapy–current status and future directions. Precision Radiation Oncology. 2022;**6**(2):164-176

[56] Paganetti H, editor. Proton Therapy Physics. 2nd ed. Boca Raton: CRC Press; 2018. DOI: 10.1201/b22053. eBook. ISBN 9781315228310

[57] Bentzen SM, Constine LS, Deasy JO, Eisbruch A, Jackson A, Marks LB, et al. Quantitative analyses of Normal tissue effects in the clinic (QUANTEC): An introduction to the scientific issues. International Journal of

Radiation Oncology, Biology, Physics. 2010;**76**(3):S3-S9

[58] Jd C. Toxicity criteria of the radiation therapy oncology group (RTOG) and the European organization for research and treatment of cancer (EORTC). International Journal of Radiation Oncology, Biology, Physics. 1995;**31**:1341-1346

[59] Marks LB, Yorke ED, Jackson A, Ten Haken RK, Constine LS, Eisbruch A, et al. Use of normal tissue complication probability models in the clinic. International Journal of Radiation Oncology, Biology, Physics. 2010;**76**(3):S10-S19

[60] Fager M, Toma-Dasu I, Kirk M, Dolney D, Diffenderfer ES, Vapiwala N, et al. Linear energy transfer painting with proton therapy: A means of reducing radiation doses with equivalent clinical effectiveness. International Journal of Radiation Oncology, Biology, Physics. 2015;**91**(5):1057-1064

[61] MacDonald SM, Patel SA, Hickey S, Specht M, Isakoff SJ, Gadd M, et al. Proton therapy for breast cancer after mastectomy: Early outcomes of a prospective clinical trial. International Journal of Radiation Oncology, Biology, Physics. 2013;**86**(3):484-490

[62] Dutz A, Agolli L, Baumann M, Troost EG, Krause M, Hölscher T, et al. Early and late side effects, dosimetric parameters and quality of life after proton beam therapy and IMRT for prostate cancer: A matched-pair analysis. Acta Oncologica. 2019;**58**(6):916-925

[63] Classen J, Belka C, Paulsen F, Budach W, Hoffmann W, Bamberg M. Radiation-induced gastrointestinal toxicity. Pathophysiology, approaches to treatment and prophylaxis. Strahlentherapie und Onkologie: Organ

der Deutschen Rontgengesellschaft...
[et al]. 1998;**174**:82-84

[64] Liang X, Bradley JA,
Zheng D, Rutenberg M, Yeung D,
Mendenhall N, et al. Prognostic factors
of radiation dermatitis following
passive-scattering proton therapy for
breast cancer. Radiation Oncology.
2018;**13**(1):1-8

[65] Arimura T, Ogino T, Yoshiura T,
Toi Y, Kawabata M, Chuman I, et al.
Effect of film dressing on acute radiation
dermatitis secondary to proton beam
therapy. International Journal of
Radiation Oncology, Biology, Physics.
2016;**95**(1):472-476

[66] Vennarini S, Del Baldo G,
Lorentini S, Pertile R, Fabozzi F, Merli P,
et al. Acute hematological toxicity during
cranio-spinal proton therapy in pediatric
brain embryonal tumors. Cancers.
2022;**14**(7):1653

[67] Song S, Park HJ, Yoon JH, Kim DW,
Park J, Shin D, et al. Proton beam
therapy reduces the incidence of acute
haematological and gastrointestinal
toxicities associated with craniospinal
irradiation in pediatric brain tumors.
Acta Oncologica. 2014;**53**(9):1158-1164

[68] Langendijk JA, Lambin P,
De Ruysscher D, Widder J, Bos M,
Verheij M. Selection of patients for
radiotherapy with protons aiming at
reduction of side effects: The model-
based approach. Radiotherapy and
Oncology. 2013;**107**(3):267-273

[69] Jones B, McMahon SJ, Prise KM.
The radiobiology of proton therapy:
Challenges and opportunities around
relative biological effectiveness. Clinical
Oncology. 2018;**30**(5):285-292

[70] Rana S, Bennouna J,
Samuel EJ, Gutierrez AN. Development

and long-term stability of a
comprehensive daily QA program for
a modern pencil beam scanning (PBS)
proton therapy delivery system. Journal
of Applied Clinical Medical Physics.
2019;**20**(4):29-44

[71] Hoffmann A, Oborn B,
Moteabbed M, Yan S, Bortfeld T,
Knopf A, et al. MR-guided proton
therapy: A review and a preview.
Radiation Oncology. 2020;**15**(1):1-3

[72] Ming X, Wang W, Shahnazi K,
Sun J, Zhang Q, Li P, et al. Dosimetric
comparison between carbon, proton
and photon radiation for renal
retroperitoneal soft tissue sarcoma
recurrence or metastasis after radical
nephrectomy. International Journal of
Radiation Biology. 2022;**98**(2):183-190

[73] Thomas H, Timmermann B.
Paediatric proton therapy. The
British Journal of Radiology.
2020;**93**(1107):20190601

[74] Nathan YY, DeWees TA, Voss MM,
Breen WG, Chiang JS, Ding JX, et al.
Cardiopulmonary toxicity following
intensity-modulated proton therapy
(IMPT) versus intensity-modulated
radiation therapy (IMRT) for stage III
non-small cell lung cancer. Clinical Lung
Cancer. 2022;**23**(8):e526-e535

[75] Kim C, Kim YJ, Lee N, Ahn SH,
Kim KH, Kim H, et al. Evaluation
of the dosimetric effect of scattered
protons in clinical practice in passive
scattering proton therapy. Journal
of Applied Clinical Medical Physics.
2021;**22**(6):104-118

[76] Bahn E, Bauer J, Harrabi S,
Herfarth K, Debus J, Alber M. Late
contrast enhancing brain lesions in
proton-treated patients with low-
grade glioma: Clinical evidence for
increased periventricular sensitivity and

variable RBE. International Journal of Radiation Oncology, Biology, Physics. 2020;**107**(3):571-578

[77] Onorato G, Di Schiavi E, Di Cunto F. Understanding the effects of deep space radiation on nervous system: The role of genetically tractable experimental models. Frontiers in Physics. 2020;**8**:362

[78] Xiang M, Chang DT, Pollom EL. Second cancer risk after primary cancer treatment with three-dimensional conformal, intensity-modulated, or proton beam radiation therapy. Cancer. 2020;**126**(15):3560-3568

[79] Uezono H, Indelicato DJ, Rotondo RL, Vega RB, Bradfield SM, Morris CG, et al. Treatment outcomes after proton therapy for Ewing sarcoma of the pelvis. International Journal of Radiation Oncology, Biology, Physics. 2020;**107**(5):974-981

[80] Greenberger BA, Yock TI. The role of proton therapy in pediatric malignancies: Recent advances and future directions. Seminars in Oncology. New York: Grune & Stratton; 2020;**47**(1):8-22. DOI: 10.1053/j. seminoncol.2020.02.002. ISSN: 093-7754

[81] Vapiwala N, Wong JK, Handorf E, Paly J, Grewal A, Tendulkar R, et al. A pooled toxicity analysis of moderately hypofractionated proton beam therapy and intensity modulated radiation therapy in early-stage prostate cancer patients. International Journal of Radiation Oncology, Biology, Physics. 2021;**110**(4):1082-1089

[82] De Marzi L, Patriarca A, Scher N, Thariat J, Vidal M. Exploiting the full potential of proton therapy: An update on the specifics and innovations towards spatial or temporal optimisation of dose delivery. Cancer/Radiothérapie. 2020;**24**(6-7):691-698

[83] Kutcher GJ, Burman C, Brewster L, Goitein M, Mohan R. Histogram reduction method for calculating complication probabilities for three-dimensional treatment planning evaluations. International Journal of Radiation Oncology, Biology, Physics. 1991;**21**(1):137-146

[84] Joiner MC, van der Kogel A. Basic Clinical Radiobiology. 4th ed. London: CRC Press; 2009. DOI: 10.1201/b15450. ISBN: 9780429190896

[85] Bhatia S, Armenian SH, Armstrong GT, van Dulmen-den Broeder E, Hawkins MM, Kremer LC, et al. Collaborative research in childhood Cancer survivorship: The current landscape. Journal of Clinical Oncology : Official Journal of the American Society of Clinical Oncology. 2015;**33**(27):3055-3064

[86] Ladra MM, Szymonifka JD, Mahajan A, Friedmann AM, Yong Yeap B, Goebel CP, et al. Preliminary results of a phase II trial of proton radiotherapy for pediatric rhabdomyosarcoma. Journal of Clinical Oncology : Official Journal of the American Society of Clinical Oncology. 2014;**32**(33):3762-3770

[87] Greenberger BA, Pulsifer MB, Ebb DH, MacDonald SM, Jones RM, Butler WE, et al. Clinical outcomes and late endocrine, neurocognitive, and visual profiles of proton radiation for pediatric low-grade gliomas. International Journal of Radiation Oncology, Biology, Physics. 2014;**89**(5):1060-1068

[88] Jimenez RB, Sethi R, Depauw N, Pulsifer MB, Adams J, McBride SM, et al. Proton radiation therapy for pediatric

medulloblastoma and supratentorial primitive neuroectodermal tumors: Outcomes for very young children treated with upfront chemotherapy. International Journal of Radiation Oncology, Biology, Physics. 2013;**87**(1):120-126

[89] Chung CS, Yock TI, Nelson K, Xu Y, Keating NL, Tarbell NJ. Incidence of second malignancies among patients treated with proton versus photon radiation. International Journal of Radiation Oncology, Biology, Physics. 2013;**87**(1):46-52

[90] Lomax AJ, Böhringer T, Bolsi A, Coray D, Emert F, Goitein G, et al. Treatment planning and verification of proton therapy using spot scanning: Initial experiences. Medical Physics. 2004;**31**(11):3150-3157

[91] Favaudon V, Caplier L, Monceau V, Pouzoulet F, Sayarath M, Fouillade C, et al. Ultrahigh dose-rate FLASH irradiation increases the differential response between normal and tumor tissue in mice. Science Translational Medicine. 2014;**6**(245):245ra93

[92] Vozenin MC, De Fornel P, Petersson K, Favaudon V, Jaccard M, Germond JF, et al. The advantage of FLASH radiotherapy confirmed in Mini-pig and Cat-cancer patients. Clinical Cancer Research : An Official Journal of the American Association for Cancer Research. 2019;**25**(1):35-42

[93] Durante M, Orecchia R, Loeffler JS. Charged-particle therapy in cancer: Clinical uses and future perspectives. Nature Reviews. Clinical Oncology. 2017;**14**(8):483-495

[94] Baumann BC, Mitra N, Harton JG, Xiao Y, Wojcieszynski AP, Gabriel PE, et al. Comparative effectiveness of proton vs photon therapy as part of concurrent chemoradiotherapy for locally advanced cancer. JAMA Oncology. 2020;**6**(2):237-246

[95] Barker HE, Paget JT, Khan AA, Harrington KJ. The tumour microenvironment after radiotherapy: Mechanisms of resistance and recurrence. Nature Reviews. Cancer. 2015;**15**(7):409-425

[96] Gandhi SJ, Minn AJ, Vonderheide RH, Wherry EJ, Hahn SM, Maity A. Awakening the immune system with radiation: Optimal dose and fractionation. Cancer Letters. 2015;**368**(2):185-190

[97] Galluzzi L, Buqué A, Kepp O, Zitvogel L, Kroemer G. Immunological effects of conventional chemotherapy and targeted anticancer agents. Cancer Cell. 2015;**28**(6):690-714

Chapter 4

Single Ionization of Methane Molecule by Directive Proton Impact: High Energies Domain

Mohammed Sahlaoui, Abdel Karim Ferouani
and Abdessamad Sekkal

Abstract

The aim of this work is to give a simple and precise theoretical formalism to study the single ionization of small molecular targets by swift proton impact. The mathematical formalism given here for the sake to calculate the differential cross sections is based on the first-Born approximation using the Coulomb wave function. The incident and scattered continuum states of the proton are described by plane wave functions, and the ejected electron is described by a Coulomb wave function. The formalism under consideration is applied to study the single ionization of methane molecule. The comparison between our results and the experimental data showed good agreement.

Keywords: cross section, first-born approximation, coulomb wave function, single ionization by proton impact, methane molecule

1. Introduction

The study of ionization processes of atomic and molecular targets by impact of charged particles is actually considered as an important field of research, since the process is found in several domains of modern physics such as plasma physics, radiation physics, astrophysics, radiotherapy and planetary atmospheres [1, 2]. The interaction of charged particles with atomic and molecular targets leads to this kind of ionization reaction. In atomic and molecular collision theory, the analysis of the single ionization process constitutes an excellent tool to understand the structure of matter and the dynamics of atoms and molecules as well as the mechanism of the reaction. In addition, knowledge of total or differential cross sections in energy and angle plays an essential role to give substantial information of different ionization processes in many applications, for example, in astronomy [3, 4], medicine and biology [5, 6], irradiation of living matter [7, 8] and in cancer treatment [9]. Depending on the nature of the ionization process, we often need the corresponding mathematical formalisms to extract precise results based on accurate numerical calculations. However, the implementation of mathematical calculations is often complicated and the corresponding numerical codes prove to be very complex to realize. The majority of problems that appear during the mathematical calculations arise from the several interactions between the different particles. Regarding the numerical programing, in fact, it could be very complicated to write an optimized and accurate numerical code, as we often deal with complicated mathematical formulas and special functions in the complex space may be with contour integrals and complex singularities. The computation time is also a very important factor to obtain in-depth information. We frequently evade these problems by simplifying the mathematical formalism using theoretical and numerical approximations. So, the researcher has to choose the necessary approximations to make the calculations manageable, on the condition that the formalism gives good information on the nature of the process under study.

In the literature, we can find several theoretical and experimental studies of the ionization process by charged particles impact. These studies have been performed on atomic targets and developed to deal with molecular targets. In the experimental side, Langmuir and Jones (1928) [10], carried out the first work on simple ionization by electron impact of N_2 and H_2 molecules, quickly followed by those of Rudberg in 1930 [11]. Subsequently, no work would deal with this aspect of the research until the end of the sixties, where Ehrhardt et al. [12] and Amaldi et al. [13] have studied, respectively, the two electrons coincidence of the ionization reaction of helium and a thin film of carbon by electron impact. On the other hand, Bethe [14], then Massey and Mohr [15], have given series of works in the theoretical domain. They succeeded in establishing the theoretical bases to describe the ionization process using Born approximation to calculate cross sections. In 1932, Hughes and McMillen [15] measured total, simply and doubly differentials cross sections of the ionization of argon atom by electron impact [16]. In 1960, Peterkop [17] then Rudge and Seaton (1964, 1965) contributed by giving theoretical formulations of the single ionization problem, by proposing several approximations to study the collision problem as three-body systems. They were the first to establish the concept of the effective charge as a function of momentum vectors of the scattered and ejected electrons in the so called (e,2e) reaction. This would make it possible, not only to simplify the study of the ionization reaction but also to make it possible to describe the post-collision reaction between the outgoing particles [18].

Several works have been interested to the interaction of the CH_4 molecule with charged particles such as ions, electrons, positrons and protons [19–20]. Most of these works are focused on the calculations of total and differential cross sections of the simple ionization of this molecule by electron impact. We can remark that, studies of the simple ionization of the molecule by proton impact are extremely rare. However, we can find the important works of: Senger [21] who measured the double differential cross section (DDCS) for proton projectile of energies from 0.25 to 2.0 MeV, Tachino et al. [22] that use the continuum distorted wave-eikonal initial state approximation (CDW-EIS) to calculate the DDCS for 2.0 MeV proton impact for different energies for the ejected electron. The contribution that we want to give here, is a study of the simple ionization of methane molecule by proton impact using the first-Born approximation 1 Coulomb wave model (FBA-CW) without and with Salin factor to take into account the transition to the continuum of the active electron. In this model, the incident and scattered proton are described by plane wave functions, whereas the ejected electron is described by a simple Coulomb wave function. This model has been used to study the single ionization of the water molecule by electron impact [23] where the model proves his power to give accurate results in the high energies domain with less difficulty in numerical computations. In this model, we use the description of Moccia for the molecular wave function where the ground state of methane molecule is described as an expansion over Slater type basis [24], centered on the carbon atom.

The objective of our work consists on studying the simple ionization of methane molecule by directive proton impact. Understanding this reaction is very important to study the different reaction in living mater and plasmas. This is because the molecule under consideration forms an important component in biological tissue and in certain planetary atmospheres, interstellar medium and even for medical considerations (see for example: [7, 25]).

2. Theoretical background

The simple ionization process of an atomic or molecular target by proton impact can be explained by the following **Figure 1**.

The **Figure 1** above gives a simple representation for the simple ionization of atomic or molecular target by proton impact. This process can also be presented in the following equation:

$$p(E_i, \mathbf{k}_i) + T(w_i) \rightarrow p(E_s, \mathbf{k}_s) + T^+(w_f) + e^-(E_e, \mathbf{k}_e) \tag{1}$$

where:

$T(w_i)$: the atomic or molecular target in the initial energy w_i.

$T^+(w_f)$: the atomic or molecular residual ion in the final energy w_f.

$p(\mathbf{k}_i)$: the incident proton with the momentum vector $\mathbf{k}_i$ and energy E_i.

$p(\mathbf{k}_s)$: the scattered proton with the momentum vector $\mathbf{k}_s$ and energy E_s.

$e^-(\mathbf{k}_e)$: the ejected electron with the momentum vector $\mathbf{k}_e$ and energy E_e.

In a collision reaction, kinematic constraints are the conservation of the energy and the momentum:

$$E_i + w_i = E_s + E_e + w_f + E_r \quad \text{and} \quad \mathbf{k}_i = \mathbf{k}_s + \mathbf{k}_e + \mathbf{Q} \tag{2}$$

Or

$$E_i = E_s + E_e + E_r + IP \quad \text{and} \quad \mathbf{k}_i = \mathbf{k}_s + \mathbf{k}_e + \mathbf{Q} \tag{3}$$

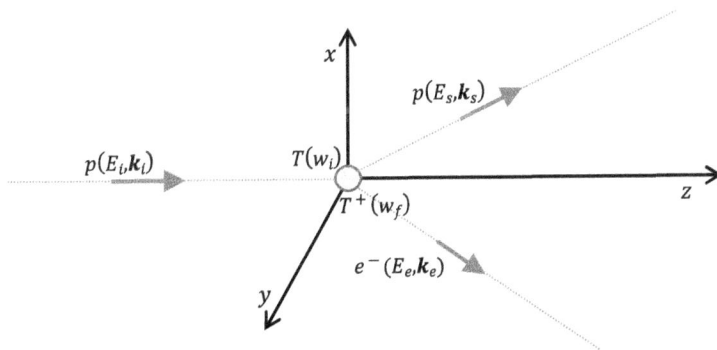

Figure 1.
The simple ionization process.

Where $PI = w_f - w_i$ represents the ionization energy of the active electron and E_r and Q are the recoil energy and recoil momentum of the ion. The first equation in (2) can be written as:

$$\frac{k_i^2}{2\mu} = \frac{k_s^2}{2\mu} + \frac{k_e^2}{2} + \frac{Q^2}{2M} + IP \tag{4}$$

μ is the proton mass and M is the target mass. In the case of high incident energies, we generally have high scattering energies and the momentum Q is very small compared to the momentums k_s and k_e and as the target is very heavy ($M \gg$) compared to the free particles (one proton is about 1837 times heavier than an electron) the recoil energy $E_r = Q^2/(2M)$ is often neglected. This is why in the literature we found **Eq. (3)** written in the form:

$$E_i = E_s + E_e + IP \quad \text{and} \quad k_i = k_s + k_e + Q \tag{5}$$

The triple differential cross section (TDCS) that measures the probability for an incident proton with the energy E_i and the momentum k_i excites a target electron to the continuum with the energy E_e and momentum k_e, and the proton scatter with the energy E_s and momentum k_e is defined as:

$$\frac{d^3\sigma}{dk_s dk_e dE_e} = \frac{k_e k_s}{k_i} S(s) \left| \langle \psi_f | V | \psi_i \rangle \right|^2 \delta(E_i - E_s - E_e + IP) \tag{6}$$

Where $\delta(x)$ is the delta function and $S(s)$ is Salin factor to take into account the transition to the continuum of the active electron:

$$S(s) = \frac{s}{1 - \exp(-s)}; \quad s = \frac{2\pi\mu}{|k_i - \mu k_e|} \tag{7}$$

The TDCS is most sensitive test for the single ionization process, since it is a physical quantity that gives a complete description over the kinematic of the ionization process.

In the present work, the target under consideration is the CH_4 molecule ionized by proton impact:

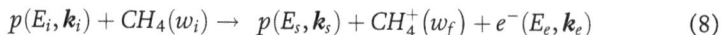

$$p(E_i, k_i) + CH_4(w_i) \rightarrow p(E_s, k_s) + CH_4^+(w_f) + e^-(E_e, k_e) \tag{8}$$

In atomic unit we have:

$$k_i^2 = 2\mu E_i \quad , \quad k_s^2 = 2\mu E_s \quad and \quad k_e^2 = 2E_e \tag{9}$$

If we are interested to the ejected particle, the double differential cross section (DDCS) can be deduced from the TDCS by integration over the scattering solid angle $\hat{k}_s$:

$$\frac{d^{(2)}\sigma}{dk_e dE_e} = \int d\hat{k}_s \frac{d^{(3)}\sigma}{dk_s d\hat{k}_e dE_e} \tag{10}$$

In **Eq. (6)**, V represents the interaction potential energy:

$$V = \sum_{j=1}^{N} \frac{Z_j}{|\boldsymbol{r}_0 - \boldsymbol{R}_j|} - \sum_{i=1}^{n} \frac{1}{|\boldsymbol{r}_0 - \boldsymbol{r}_i|} \tag{11}$$

Where Z_j is the charge of the nuclei j, r_i is the position vector of the ith electron of the molecular target, R_j is the position vector of the jth nuclei. The initial and final states can be written in the following forms:

$$|\psi_i\rangle = |\phi_i(\boldsymbol{k}_i, \boldsymbol{r}_0)\varphi_i(\boldsymbol{r}_1, \boldsymbol{r}_2, \cdots, \boldsymbol{r}_n)\rangle \tag{12}$$

$$|\psi_f\rangle = |\phi_s(\boldsymbol{k}_s, \boldsymbol{r}_0)\varphi_f(\boldsymbol{r}_1, \boldsymbol{r}_2, \cdots, \boldsymbol{r}_n)\rangle \tag{13}$$

$\phi_i(\boldsymbol{k}_i, \boldsymbol{r}_0)$ and $\phi_s(\boldsymbol{k}_s, \boldsymbol{r}_0)$ are the wave functions of the incident and scattered proton chosen here as plane wave functions $\exp(i\,\boldsymbol{k}_i \cdot \boldsymbol{r}_0)$ and $\exp(i\,\boldsymbol{k}_s \cdot \boldsymbol{r}_0)$. Now if we use the so-called frozen core approximation (FCA), we can reduce the initial and final states to the following forms:

$$|\psi_i\rangle = |\phi_i(\boldsymbol{k}_i, \boldsymbol{r}_0)\varphi_i(\boldsymbol{r}_1)\rangle \tag{14}$$

$$|\psi_f\rangle = |\phi_s(\boldsymbol{k}_s, \boldsymbol{r}_0)\varphi_f(\boldsymbol{r}_1)\rangle \tag{15}$$

where only the active electron is considered, and we can reduce the potential energy to

$$V = \frac{1}{r_0} - \frac{1}{|\boldsymbol{r}_0 - \boldsymbol{r}_1|} \tag{16}$$

The molecular electrons are distributed among the five orbitals $1A_1$, $2A_1$, $1T_{2x}$, $1T_{2y}$ and $1T_{2z}$. If the reference origin is chosen on the carbon nuclei, each molecular orbital can be defined by linear combinations of Slater-type functions centered over the carbon atom [4]:

$$\varphi_i(\boldsymbol{r}_1) = \sum_{k=1}^{N_i} a_{ik} \Phi_{n_{ik}l_{ik}m_{ik}}^{\xi_{ik}}(\boldsymbol{r}_1) \tag{17}$$

a_{ik} is the contribution magnitude of the basis element $\Phi_{n_{ik}l_{ik}m_{ik}}^{\xi_{ik}}(\boldsymbol{r}_1)$ given in the molecular frame, as follows:

$$\Phi_{n_{ik}l_{ik}m_{ik}}^{\xi_{ik}}(\boldsymbol{r}_1) = R_{n_{ik}}^{\xi_{ik}}(r_1) S_{l_{ik},m_{ik}}(\hat{r}_1) \tag{18}$$

$R_{n_{ik}}^{\xi_{ik}}(r_1)$ is the radial part chosen as a Slater function and $S_{l_{ik},m_{ik}}(\hat{r}_1)$ is the real spherical harmonic,

$$\begin{cases} S_{l_{ik},m_{ik}}(\hat{r}_1) = \left(\frac{m_{ik}}{2|m_{ik}|}\right)^{\frac{-1}{2}} \left\{ Y_{l_{ik}-|m_{ik}|}(\hat{r}_1) + (-1)^{m_{ik}} \left(\frac{m_{ik}}{|m_{ik}|}\right) Y_{l_{ik}|m_{ik}|}(\hat{r}_1) \right\} \\ S_{l_{ik}\,0}(\hat{r}_1) = Y_{l_{ik}0}(\hat{r}_1) \end{cases} \tag{19}$$

The molecular wave function given in **Eq. (17)** is defined in a molecular reference frame; we need then to transform it to the laboratory reference frame. This transformation is possible thanks to the relationship:

$$Y_{l_{ik},m_{ik}}(\hat{r}_1) = \sum_{\mu=-l_{ik}}^{l_{ik}} D^{l_{ik}}_{\mu_{ik},m_{ik}}(\alpha,\beta,\gamma) Y_{l_{ik},\mu_{ik}}(\hat{r}_1) \tag{20}$$

Where $D^{l_{ik}}_{\mu_{ik},m_{ik}}(\alpha,\beta,\gamma)$ is a rotation operator, α, β and γ are the Euler angles. Because the target is randomly orientated, the measured cross section is an average over all possible orientations. This is why we need to average the theoretical cross section over all the Euler angles:

$$\frac{d^{(2)}\bar{\sigma}}{d\hat{k}_e dE_e} = \frac{1}{8\pi} \int d\beta \sin\beta d\alpha \, d\gamma \, \frac{d^{(2)}\sigma}{d\hat{k}_e dE_e} \tag{21}$$

In the present formalism, the ejected electron is described by a Coulomb wave function.

$$\varphi_f(k_e, r_1) = \exp\left(\frac{\pi}{k_e}\right)\Gamma\left(1+\frac{i}{k_e}\right){}_1F_1\left[\frac{-i}{k_e}, 1, -i(k_e \cdot r_1 + k_e r_1)\right]\exp(ik_e \cdot r_1) \tag{22}$$

where the effective ionic charge is taken equal to 1.

3. Results and discussion

In **Figures 2** and **3**, we present the results concerning the angular distribution of the DDCS for the simple ionization of CH_4 molecule by proton impact. The incident energy is $E_i = 2$ **MeV**, a very high energy in addition to the fact that proton mass is very large compared to the electron one, which justifies the choice of the first Born approximation as a good model in this case. Several results of the DDCS are extracted for ejection energies $E_e = 11.3$ **eV**, 20 eV, 50 eV, 100 eV, 200 eV and 1000 eV. Furthermore, the incidence energy $E_i = 2$ **MeV** indicates that the time of the collision reaction is very short, we deal then with a very fast collision reaction which justifies that the FCA can be safely used [26]. In the goal to verify the formalism and the numerical code, our results extracted by the FBA-CW model are compared to the theoretical results of Tachino et al. [22] obtained by the CDW-EIS model and to the experimental data found in the paper of Senger [21] (in this paper Senger used the experimental data of Lynch and para [27]). In our numerical calculations of the DDCS, the description Moccia [19] for the molecular wave function is used for meth-ane molecule. We recalled that in this description each molecular orbital is expanded over a Slater-type basis centered on the carbon atom under the assumption that this atom is the heaviest compared to hydrogen atoms.

In **Figures 2** and **3**, the DDCS results are presented in logarithmic scales (left side) and linear scales (right side) in order to have a clear view of the difference between the theoretical models. In these figures, our results are also presented with and with-out Salin factor (see **Eq. (8)** of **(6)**) to demonstrate the effect of this factor on the cross section, or in other terms to clearly see the effect of the transfer to the contin-uum of the active electron. Generally speaking, from the comparison between our results and the experimental data, we can notice a good agreement between them for the ejection energies from 100 eV to 1000 eV, and an acceptable agreement for energies 20 eV and 50 eV. We also clearly observe that our results are close to the

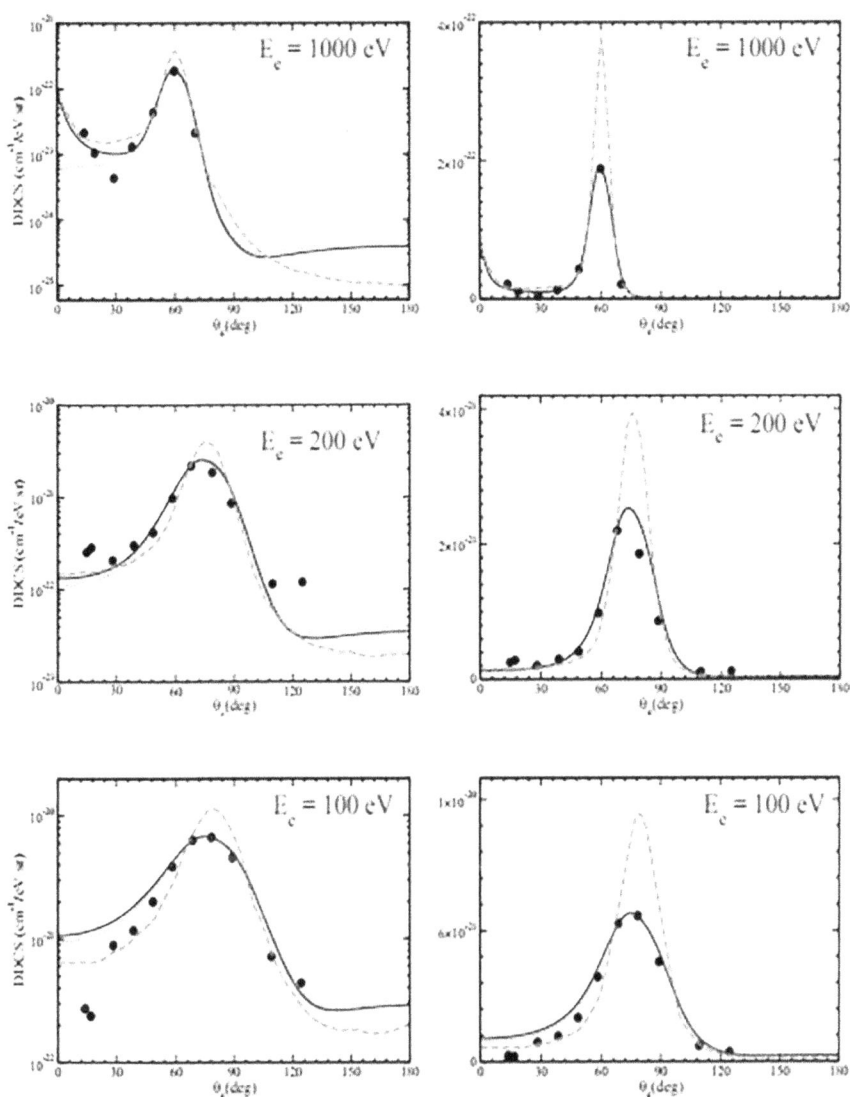

Figure 2.
Angular distribution of the DDCS of the simple ionization of CH_4 molecule by proton impact of $E_i = 2$ MeV for different ejection energies E_e. Solid and dotted lines are, respectively, our results from the FBA-CW model with and without Salin factor. Dashed line: the results of Tachino et al. [22] given from the CDW-EIS model. Solid circles: the experimental data [21]. left in logarithmic scale and right in linear scale.

experimental data in the peaks compared to theoretical results of Tachino et al. [22] obtained from the CDW-EIS model.

Concerning the results where the ejection energy $E_i = 11.3$ eV, we can clearly see that our formalism and that of Tachino et al. [22] cannot correctly describe the collision reaction for this scale of ejection energy or for lower energies. We believe that when the electron leaves the molecule with a low velocity, it will undergo different interactions, such as the distortion of the wave function due to the interaction with the residual ion and the interaction with the proton. We also think that there are

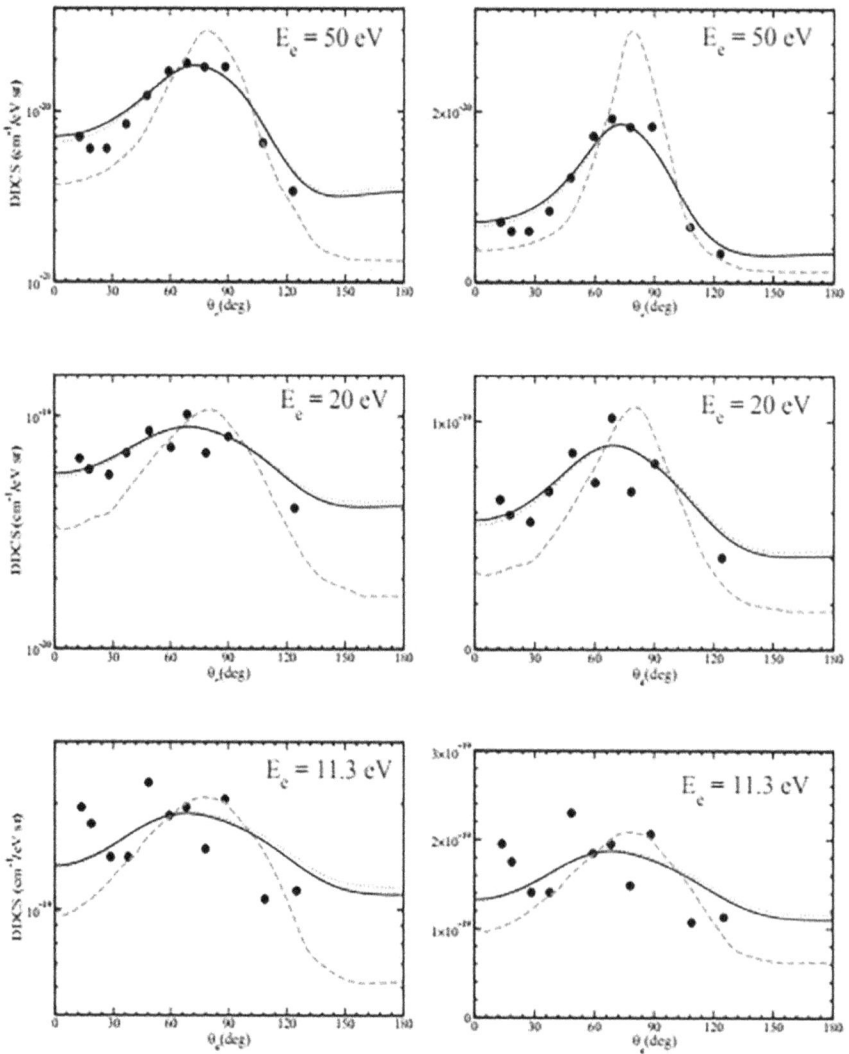

Figure 3.
The same as in Figure 2.

many transitions of the active electron from the intermediate state before to be ejected, which requires calculations of the transition amplitude with another model that takes in to account this kind of transitions or use higher orders Born approximation.

Contrary to the numerical computation of the TDCS, the computation time of the DDCS is very important; this is why in the work of Tachino et al. [22] where the CDW-EIS model is used, the molecular wave function was truncated by excluding the contribution of Slater type orbitals of principle number $n \geq 7$. In the work of Tachino et al. [22], as in ours, the wave function of the CH_4 molecule is described using the Slater type basis given by Moccia [19]. However, in our formalism, all the elements of this basis are used to compute the DDCS. For the purpose to study the truncation

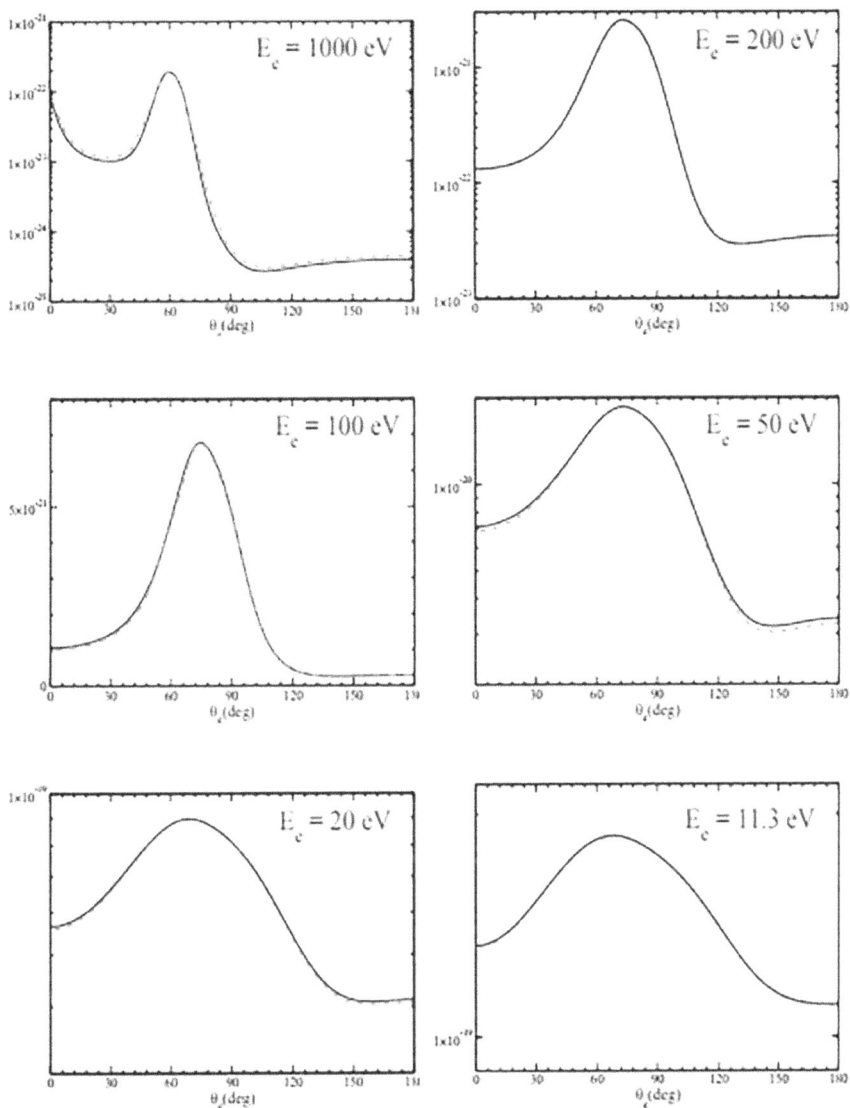

Figure 4.
The DDCS of single ionization of CH_4 by proton impact of $E_i = 2$ MeV for different ejection energies E_e. Solid and dotted lines are, respectively, our results from the FBA-CW model with and without truncation of the original basis of Moccia [19] by excluding the contribution of slater type orbitals of principle number $n \geq 7$.

effect of this molecular basis on the computation accuracy, we compare in **Figure 4** our theoretical results without and with truncation by excluding the contribution of Slater type orbitals of principle number $n \geq 7$.

Tachino et al. [22] considered that in the original description of Moccia [19], the contribution of Slater type molecular orbitals of principal numbers $n \geq 7$ is negligible compared to the contribution of those of $n < 7$. From the results given in **Figure 4**, we can clearly see that there is just a very little difference between the curves with and without truncation. This ensures that the difference between our results and those of the Tachino et al. [22] is not due to the truncation of the original description of the molecular wave function given by Moccia [19]. We can say then that our formalism of the FBA-CW model clearly gives precise results for high ejection energies compared to the CDW-EIS model used by Tachino et al. [22].

4. Conclusion

Single ionization of methane molecule by 2 MeV proton impact was considered in the present paper. The results given here are extracted using our formalism of the FBA-CW model. These theoretical data are compared to the theoretical results of Tachino et al. [22] obtained from the CDW-EIS model. All these findings are compared to the experimental data given by Senger [21]. We generally found that our results are in well agreement with the experiment and better than those of Tachino et al. [22] for high ejection energies.

This proves once more that the simple formalism that we have developed in the frame of the FBA-CW model can provide very accurate results, under certain geometric and energetic conditions. However, as any other approximated model certain corrections are needed to improve the accuracy of the formalism in high incident energies domain. For example, we can take into consideration the distortion of the ejected electron wave function. We may also take into account the capture phenomenon.

Acknowledgements

The work of Pr A K Ferouani was supported by DGRSDT, Algerian Ministry of Higher Education and Research, under Project PRFU-code A11N01EP130220230001.

Author details

Mohammed Sahlaoui[1,2], Abdel Karim Ferouani[1,2]* and Abdessamad Sekkal[3]

1 Ecole Supérieure en Sciences Appliquées de Tlemcen, Tlemcen, Algeria

2 Department of Physics, Faculty of Sciences, Theoretical Physics Laboratory, University of Tlemcen, Tlemcen, Algeria

3 Ecole Supérieure des Sciences Appliquées d'Alger, Algeria

*Address all correspondence to: ferouani_karim@yahoo.fr

IntechOpen

References

[1] Enos CS, Lee AR, Brenton AG. Electronic excitation of atmospheric molecules by proton impact. International Journal of Mass Spectrometry and Ion Processes. 1991; **104**(2):137-144. DOI: 10.1016/0168-1176 (91)80005-8

[2] Khare SP, Sharma MK, Tomar S. Electron impact ionization of methane. Journal of Physics B: Atomic, Molecular and Optical Physics. 1999;**32**(13): 3147-3156. DOI: 10.1088/0953-4075/32/13/305

[3] Katayama DH, Huffman RE, O'Bryan CL. Absorption and photoionization cross sections for H_2O and D_2O in the vacuum ultraviolet. The Journal of Chemical Physics. 1973;**59**(8): 4309-4319. DOI: 10.1063/1.1680627

[4] McDanie EW, Mitchell JBA, Rudd ME. Atomic Collisions. New York: Wiley; 1993

[5] Olivera GH, Martinez AE, Rivarola RD, Fainstein PD. Theoretical calculation of electronic stopping power of water vapor by proton impact. Radiation Research. 1995;**144**(2): 241-247. DOI: 10.2307/3579265

[6] Dingfelder M, Inokuti M, Paretzke HG. Inelastic-collision cross sections of liquid water for interactions of energetic protons. Radiation Physics and Chemistry. 2000;**59**(3):255-275. DOI: 10.1016/S0969-806X(00)00263-2

[7] Nikitaki Z, Nikolov V, Mavragani IV, Mladenov E, Mangelis A, Laskaratou DA, et al. Measurement of complex DNA damage induction and repair in human cellular systems after exposure to ionizing radiations of varying linear energy transfer (LET). Free Radical Research. 2016;**50**(sup1): S64-S78. DOI: 10.1080/10715762.2016. 1232484

[8] Meylan S, Incerti S, Karamitros M, Tang N, Bueno M, Clairand I, et al. Simulation of early DNA damage after the irradiation of a fibroblast cell nucleus using Geant4-DNA. Scientific Reports. 2017;**7**(1):11923. DOI: 10.1038/ s41598-017-11851-4

[9] Alizadeh E, Orlando TM, Sanche L. Biomolecular damage induced by ionizing radiation: The direct and indirect effects of low-energy electrons on DNA. Annual Review of Physical Chemistry. 2015;**66**:379-398. DOI: 10.1146/annurev-physchem-040513-103605

[10] Langmuir I, Jones HA. Collisions between electrons and gas molecules. Physical Review. 1928;**31**(3):357-404. DOI: 10.1103/PhysRev.31.357

[11] Rudberg E. Energy losses of electrons in nitrogen. Proceedings of the Royal Society of London. Series A, Containing Papers of a Mathematical and Physical Character. 1930;**129**(811):628-651. DOI: 10.1098/rspa.1930.0179

[12] Ehrhardt H, Jung K, Knoth G, Schlemmer P. Differential cross sections of direct single electron impact ionization. Zeitschrift für Physik D Atoms, Molecules and Clusters. 1986;**1**: 3-32. DOI: 10.1007/BF01384654

[13] Amaldi U Jr, Egidi A, Marconero R, Pizzella G. Use of a two channeltron coincidence in a new line of research in atomic physics. Review of Scientific Instruments. 1969;**40**(8):1001-1004

[14] Bethe H. Zur theorie des durchgangs schneller korpuskularstrahlen durch

materie. Annalen der Physik. 1930;
397(3):325-400. DOI: 10.1002/
andp.19303970303

[15] Massey HSW, Mohr CBO. The collision of slow electrons with atoms. III.-the excitation and ionization of helium by electrons of moderate velocity, proceedings of the Royal Society of London. Series A, Containing Papers of a Mathematical and Physical Character. 1933;**140**(842):613-636. DOI: 10.1098/rspa.1933.0092

[16] Hughes AL, McMillen JH. Inelastic and elastic electron scattering in argon. Physical Review. 1932;**39**(4):585-600. DOI: 10.1103/PhysRev.39.585

[17] Peterkop RK. Asymptotic expansion of charged particles wavefunction. Latvijas PSR Zinatnu Akademijas Vestis. 1960;**9**:79-84

[18] Rudge MRH, Seaton MJ. Ionization of atomic hydrogen by electron impact, proceedings of the Royal Society of London. Series A. Mathematical and Physical Sciences. 1965;**283**(1393): 262-290. DOI: 10.1098/rspa.1965.0020

[19] Moccia R, One-Center Basis Set SCF MO's. I. HF, CH_4, and SiH_4. The Journal of Chemical Physics. 1964;**40**(8):2164-2176. DOI: 10.1063/ 1.1725489

[20] Sahlaoui M, Lasri B, Bouamoud M. Analytical formula for electron-impact ionization cross section in the one coulomb wave model. Canadian Journal of Physics. 2014;**92**(2):136-140. DOI: 10.1139/cjp-2013-0342

[21] Senger B. Calculated molecular double-differential cross-sections for ionisation under proton impact. Zeitschrift Für Physik D Atoms, Molecules and Clusters. 1988;**9**:79-89. DOI: 10.1007/BF01384450

[22] Tachino CA, Monti JM, Fojon OA, Champion C, Rivarola RD. Single electron ionization of NH_3 and CH_4 by swift proton impact. In Journal of Physics: Conference Series. 2015;**583**(1): 012020. DOI: 10.1088/1742-6596/583/1/ 012020

[23] Sahlaoui M, Bouamoud M. Cross sections for electron-impact ionization of water molecules. Canadian Journal of Physics. 2011;**89**(6):723-727. DOI: 10.1139/p11-048

[24] Sahlaoui M, Bouamoud M, Lasri B, Dogan M. Ionization of a water molecule by electron impact in coplanar symmetric and asymmetric geometries. Journal of Physics B: Atomic, Molecular and Optical Physics. 2013;**46**(11):115206. DOI: 10.1088/0953-4075/46/11/115206

[25] Wilson EH, Atreya SK. Current state of modeling the photochemistry of Titan's mutually dependent atmosphere and ionosphere. Journal of Geophysical Research: Planets. 2004;**109**:E06002. DOI: 10.1029/2003JE002181

[26] Pickett WE. Pseudopotential methods in condensed matter applications. Computer Physics Reports. 1989;**9**(3):115-197. DOI: 10.1016/ 0167-7977(89)90002-6

[27] Lynch DJ, Toburen LH, Wilson WE. Electron emission from methane, ammonia, monomethylamine, and dimethylamine by 0.25 to 2.0 MeV protons. The Journal of Chemical Physics. 1976;**64**(6):2616-2622. DOI: 10.1063/1.432515

Chapter 5

Interaction of Proton Beam with Human Tissues in Proton Therapy

Rafik Hazem

Abstract

Proton therapy is an effective and safe method to treat tumors in human body. Instead of conventional radiation (X-rays), this technique uses a heavy charged particles (protons) to treat cancer. This chapter reviews the basic aspects of the physics of proton therapy, including proton beam properties, proton interaction mechanisms, and radiation effects induced in the human tissue. A more highly conformal technique of proton therapy called "pencil beam scanning", based on intensity-modulated proton therapy (IMPT), will be also developed. The uncertainty in the determination of the relative biological effectiveness (RBE) will also be discussed in light of recent experimental results. We conclude the chapter by discussing future developments and potential challenges of proton therapy.

Keywords: proton beam, interaction mechanism, energy loss, dose-depth distribution, Bragg peak, proton therapy

1. Introduction

Following Robert Wilson's breakthrough publication "Radiological Use of Fast Protons" in 1946, which revolutionized the field of radiotherapy, proton therapy became a modality with increasing importance. Since the first treatments in the 1950s, proton beam therapy (PBT) has been increasingly used in hospital settings with similar workflows to conventional radiotherapy. Nearly 200,000 patients underwent proton beam treatment worldwide in 2020. The number of proton therapy (PT) installations will soon reach one hundred. **Figure 1** shows the increasing current treatment rooms open worldwide and those expected to open in the next few years.

Due to the favorable physical properties of protons, the use of PBT has constantly increased over the last decade. The international scientific community has made great efforts to improve the performance and effectiveness of this technology. The aim of this chapter was to report the characteristics and current developments in PBT.

2. Physical aspects

2.1 Protons interactions

When a beam of protons passes into homogeneous matter, it undergoes successive interactions with atomic electrons and nucleus. First, protons lose continuously their

63

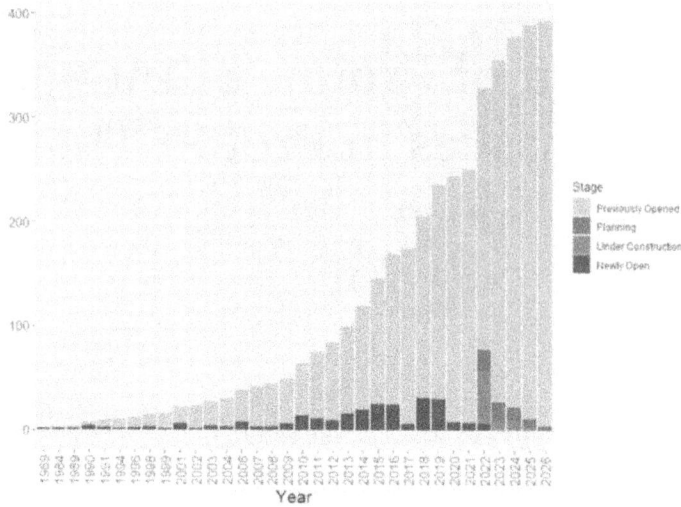

Figure 1.
Cumulative number of proton treatment rooms opened since 1964 and those projected until 2026 [1].

kinetic energy through frequent inelastic Coulomb interactions with atomic electrons (excitation and ionization of atoms). Despite these interactions, protons travel in a nearly straight line as their rest mass is much higher than that of electron (1832 times). Seeing their energy decreased, protons experience a repulsive elastic Coulombic interaction with the atomic nucleus. Due to its large mass, nucleus deflects the proton from its original straight line path. On the other hand, the non-elastic nuclear reactions between protons and the target atomic nucleus are less likely. Proton Bremsstrahlung is theoretically possible, but, at therapeutic proton beam energies, this effect is also negligible.

2.2 Protons energy loss

The energy loss of incoming protons due to inelastic Coulombic interactions with atomic electrons in the irradiated medium is described by the linear stopping power

$$S = \frac{dE}{dx} \tag{1}$$

or frequently the mass stopping power $\frac{S}{\rho} = -\frac{dE}{\rho dx}$ to make it independent of the mass density. ρ is the mass density of the material, E is the energy of the proton beam, and x is the distance. The more accurate formula of the mass stopping power that takes into account quantum mechanical effects was developed by Bloch [2]:

$$\frac{S}{\rho} = -\frac{dE}{\rho dx} = 4\pi N_A r_e^2 m_e c^2 \frac{Z}{A} \frac{z^2}{\beta^2} \left[\ln \frac{2m_e c^2 \gamma^2 \beta^2}{I} - \beta^2 - \frac{\delta}{2} - \frac{C}{Z} \right] \tag{2}$$

where N_A is the number of Avogadro, r_e is the classical radius of electron, m_e is the electron mass, z is the projectile charge, Z is the atomic number irradiated material, A is the atomic weight of irradiated material, c is light speed, $\beta = v/c$, where v is the projectile velocity, $\gamma = (1 - \beta^2)^{-1/2}$, I is the mean excitation potential of irradiated material, δ is the density corrections, and C is the shell correction item, which is important only for low energies where the particle velocity is close to that of atomic electrons. The formula shows that the proton energy loss is proportional to the inverse square of its velocity $1/v^2$. Therefore, the energy loss increases rapidly with decreasing proton velocity.

At lower energy (velocity), so in the end of its range, the proton interacts with irradiated medium through nuclear interactions. The main damage thus produced in the target is due to these interactions and it occurs in the end of proton range. This distribution of energy deposition, markedly different from that of conventional radiations, is useful for radiotherapy, as the overwhelming majority of proton energy is deposited at the end of the proton range.

We define also the Linear energy transfer (LET) as the ratio of energy transferred by a charged particle (dE) to the target atoms along its path through tissue (dx). In other words, LET is a measure of the density of ionizations along a radiation beam:

$$LET = \frac{dE}{dx} \tag{3}$$

In proton therapy, we used commonly the absorbed dose which can be calculated by the relation (4). For proton beam fluence Φ in proton/cm^2 and S/ρ in MeV/(g/cm^2), dose is calculated as:

$$D = 0.1602.\Phi.\frac{S}{\rho} \; [Gy] \tag{4}$$

2.3 Proton range

The trajectory of most protons in matter is almost linear. Therefore, the path length of the proton is almost equal to its projected range, which is an excellent approximation of range in most clinical situations. In this case, the range (R) may be calculated as:

$$R(E) = \int_{0}^{E} \left(\frac{dE}{dx}\right)^{-1} dE \tag{5}$$

2.4 Dose-depth distribution

Plotting the absorbed radiation dose versus the penetration depth of the protons, the emerged distribution is called Bragg distribution or Bragg curve (**Figure 2**).

As can be seen from the figure, the depth-dose curve for protons is characterized firstly by a low dose plateau, in the entrance region, caused predominantly by the slowly increasing energy loss with decreasing proton energy. The low absorbed energy in this region is due mainly to the electronic excitation and ionization of the target atoms. At a critical depth, the dose-depth curve experiences a distal rapid dose build-up, culminating in a maximum, and a steep fall-off at the end of their range. This behavior displayed by protons beam at the end of their path is called "Bragg peak".

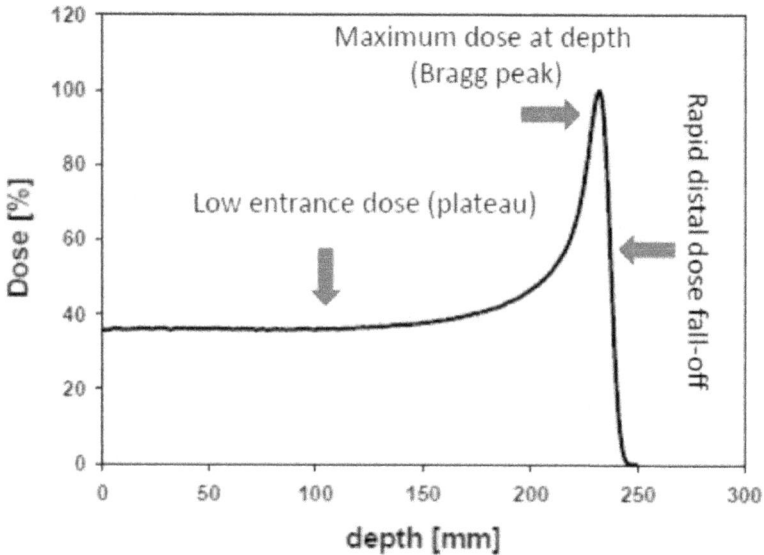

Figure 2.
Typical dose deposition as a function of depth for a proton beam.

The drastic increase of the absorbed dose occurs at low energies (velocity) of the protons, in which the nuclear interactions are predominates. In this region of few millimeters, the protons deliver the majority of their energy at the target and produce the main damage. The relative height of this "Bragg peak" is about 3–4 times the absorbed dose in the plateau.

It is worth noting that the distal fall-off in the end of the Bragg curve is very steep. In the case of 200 MeV proton beam, the fall of the peak dose from 90 to 10% occurs in about 7 mm. The depth dose distribution displayed by proton, especially the distal fall-off in the end of the dose-depth curve, has made the proton as a real candidate for the treatment of tumors in the human body. This behavior is in line with the require-ment of radiation therapy, in which researches seek to reduce the absorbed dose during the proton path in order to preserve the healthy tissues and deliver almost all of it in the tumor area. Therefore, protons can deliver a high dose to the tumor volume while sparing surrounding healthy tissues and organs at risk.

In proton beam therapy, the energetic proton travels the human tissue so fast, almost at two-thirds the speed of light, that the number of interactions in each millimeter that it travels is relatively low. So, the radiation dose absorbed by healthy tissues is relatively low. But after millions of interactions (electronic inter-actions), the proton will gradually slow down and stop. At the end of its path, when its speed is considerably reduced, the proton undergoes many more interac-tions (nuclear interactions) in a few millimeters where it deposits the majority of its energy. In this region of tumor volume (10–20 mm), the sharp energy loss results in a dramatical increase in radiation dose (high dose peak) at the end of the proton path (Bragg peak).

By varying the energy of proton beam, the Bragg peak can be moved to different depths within the patient. Knowing the Dose-depth distribution, we can know the dose maximum at the position of the tumor.

The depth of the Bragg peak is determined by the initial energy of the beam. As a prominent example of the proposed theories, Bortfeld [3] modeled the Bragg curve based on the power-law approximation where the range R_0 of protons in the medium is related to their initial energy E_0:

$$R_0 = \alpha E_0{}^P \tag{6}$$

For proton energies used in therapy (E_0 between 50 and 250 MeV), the power p was estimated to $p \approx 1.7$–1.8. Since E_0 is in MeV and R_0 in cm, the dimension of α is cm/MeV^P (p is dimensionless).

In radiotherapy, a lot of time is spent planning each treatment to ensure that the appropriate energy and dose are delivered to the tumor while minimizing the dose to normal organs as much as possible. This challenge is raised by proton therapy which has featured this particle as an appropriate candidate for radiation therapy.

3. Straggling

If all protons would lose the same amount of energy per scattering event, all would display the same range. However, the interaction of these charged particles with matter must be considered as a statistical process. Consequently, monoenergetic protons passing through matter will lose slightly different amounts of energy and will not all stop at precisely the same depth. This statistical fluctuation in the energy loss results in an uncertainty in the particle range, called "range straggling" (**Figure 3**).

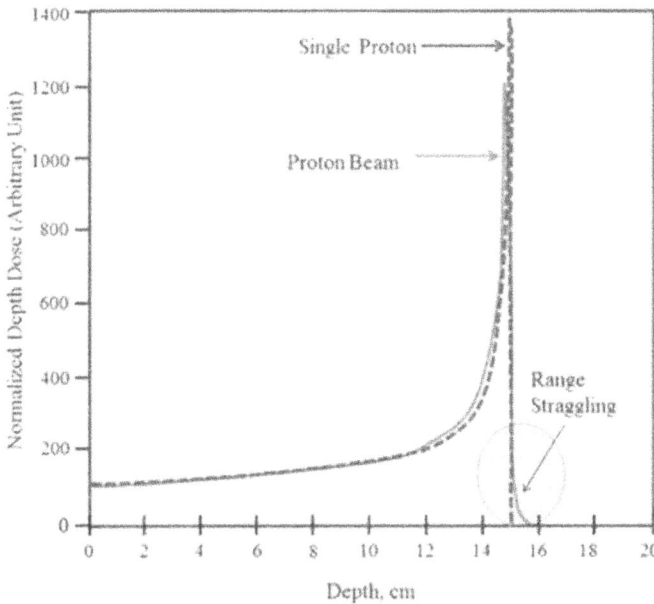

Figure 3.
Depth-dose curve of a proton beam, showing the Bragg peak and range straggling [4].

4. PBT and conventional radiations therapy

Photon therapy and proton therapy are the two main kinds of radiation therapy used in the treatment of cancer. These are different forms of ionizing radiation that work by damaging cancer cells so that they cannot reproduce and possibly die. While photons release energy along the entire path, they travel in the body, protons reserve most of energy during their path and release it where they stop in the tumor (peak Bragg) (**Figure 2**). This fundamental difference allows the proton to treat the tumor while minimizing radiation exposure to the rest of the body. Protons therefore have dosimetric characteristics different from those of conventional radiation used in radiotherapy. As indicated by **Figure 4**, after a short expansion of the absorbed dose, conventional radiation exhibits exponentially decreasing energy loss with increasing depth in medium.

In contrast, protons exhibit a plateau of low entrance dose followed by a drastic increase in energy deposition with penetration depth leading to a maximum "Bragg peak" followed by a rapid distal dose fall-off at the end of the proton range (**Figure 4**).

This magical evolution of proton energy loss with the penetration depth in matter is consistent with the requirements of radiotherapy. Indeed, effective and safe treatment of tumors inside the human body requires two conditions: sparing of normal tissue that separates the body surface from the tumor and ensures that almost all of the energy will be deposited in the tumor area. It is clear that these requirements are satisfied in the dose-depth distribution of the protons (**Figure 4**), which deliver a very low dose in the first phase of their path then release almost all of their energy at the end of their path in a well-defined position.

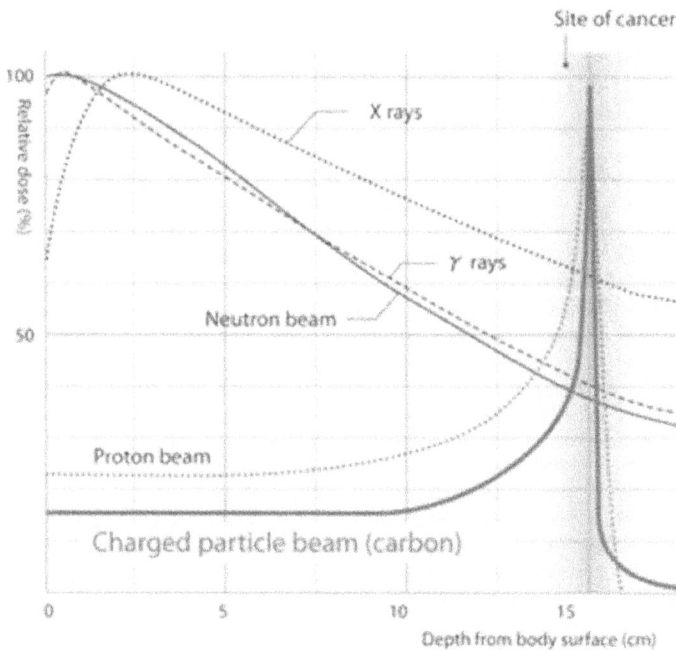

Figure 4.
Depth-dose curve of a proton, carbon ion, and other conventional radiations.

Another important advantage of the proton radiotherapy over to conventional radiation is that protons finally stop in matter, and the dose beyond the stopping position is negligible. Due to this finite range in tissue, the delivered dose in the proton radiation therapy is more sensitive to density changes, when compared to external beam photon radiation therapy. In summary, most of radiation energy of photons is deposited outside the target, while most of radiation energy of protons is deposited inside the target.

On the other hand, we know that tumors are damaged after a series of interactions between the projectile and the cancer leading to DNA breaking. They are unable to repair or copy themselves, and therefore they will die. In this way, many experts believe that protons are more successful at breaking DNA than photons [5].

5. Problems and challenges of proton therapy

So far, we have seen that protons are best suited for treating cancer with radiotherapy. But, if we consider the local extension of the tumor, proton therapy, as presented above, cannot be the suitable approach for such treatment. However, a full understanding of proton-matter interactions and a dose-depth distribution allows us to solve the two main physical problems that may arise in proton therapy: designing proton beam according to the tumor shape, and predicting the dose distribution in human tissue. To handle the mentioned problems, proton beam energy could be adjusted to reach tumor position (beam range) and shaped to conform to the tumor area. The last one is accomplished by the modulation width of the spread-out Bragg peak (SOBP).

5.1 Spread-out Bragg peak (SOBP)

The Bragg peak of monoenergetic proton beam is too narrow to cover extent of tumor volume. To produce wider depth coverage, the location of the Bragg peak can be expanded as needed using proton beams of different energies, resulting in the spread-out Bragg peak (SOBP). The SOBP is produced by superimposing Bragg peaks of different proton energies, and thereby obtaining a widened region of homogeneous dose [6–8]. This energy degrader is suitable for treating tumors at any depth (**Figure 5**).

For spreading the Bragg peak, proton therapy is generally administered through two different beam delivery systems: scattering and scanning beam delivery [9].

5.1.1 Passive scattering systems

In passive scattering mode, the narrow proton beam is laterally broadened by a scattering device and a modulator is used to generate the SOBP (**Figure 6**). A metallic filter is used to generate beam spreading with inverse square fall-off of intensity. It is then shaped using a second scatterer and collimator to provide a uniform field at the target volume. The disadvantages of this mode are significant dose delivered along the entrance path, extremely sensitive to the movements of target, and minimized integral dose.

5.1.2 Active scanning systems (pencil beam scanning)

Pencil beam scanning (the beam roughly resembles a pencil) is a more conformal proton therapy technique which is now increasingly sought after in hospitals because it allows better conformation of the absorbed dose to the tumor. Compared to other

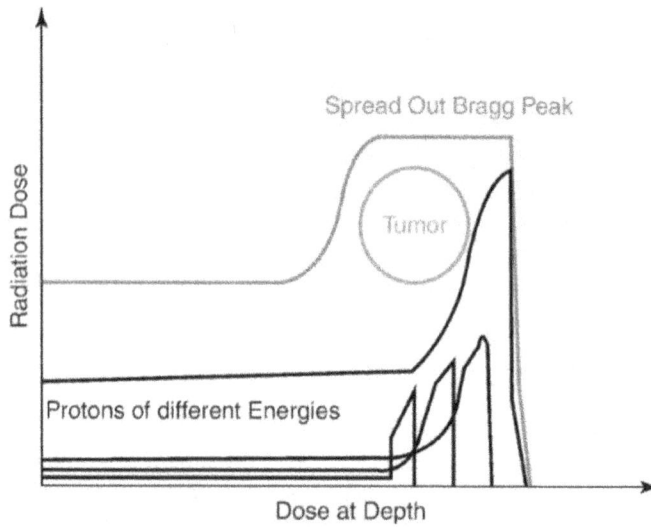

Figure 5.
Superimposition of Bragg peaks of different energies to have spread-out Bragg peak (SOBP).

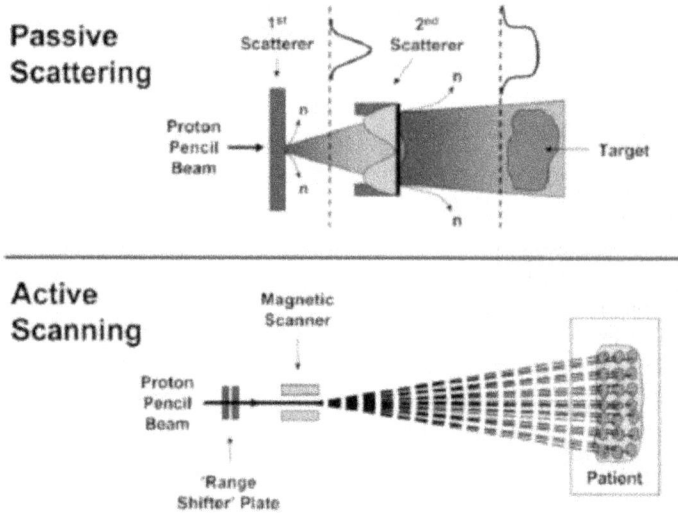

Figure 6.
Passive scattering and active scanning modes.

proton beam methods, this technique allows the proton beam to be directed so precisely to the exact desired position in the tumor where the protons release their
maximum energy dose, whereas, a lower dose is delivered to adjacent healthy tissue.
Pencil beam scanning uses magnets to steer the proton beam, creating a customized,
three-dimensional delivery shape. The target is divided into layers that are positioned
at a user-defined interval. During treatment, the dose is deposited layer by layer, from
the most distal layer to the most proximal layer sequentially. Within each layer, the
dose is deposited through individual spots that can have unique intensities and

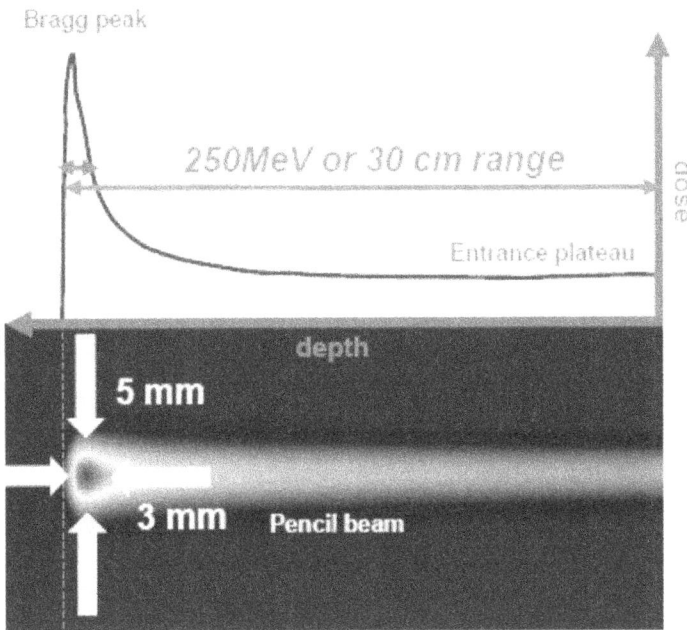

Figure 7.
Pencil beam scanning technique.

positions (**Figure 6**). Therefore, the dose is conformed to the specific shape of the tumor and destroys cancer cells while preserving critical structures nearby.

In this technique, the material present in the beam path is minimized, which will reduce beam losses and the generation of unwanted secondary particles.

The active scattering technique or pencil beam scanning has two major advantages over the passive scattering technique. First, it allows for shaping of both proximal and distal edges of the treatment field by decreasing the entry dose while maintaining absence of exit dose. Second, the neutron scatter, which is of concern regarding secondary cancer induction, is significantly reduced. On top of that, pencil beam scanning introduces the possibility of intensity-modulated proton therapy (IMPT) [10, 11].

In **Figure 7**, a narrow pencil beam of high energy ≈250 MeV at the entrance, produced by a cyclotron, is used to treat a tumor region located at 30 cm. For this energy, the Bragg peak has to occur at the same distance of the tumor and with energy variation, the user must produce a several Bragg peaks through an area of about 5×3 mm^2, which is the size of the tumor region.

6. Accelerators used in the proton therapy

The protons beam used in radiation therapy is provided by two particle accelerators, cyclotrons, and synchrotrons, which produce proton beams at typical energies between 70 and 250 MeV [12]. The cyclotron, mainly used for proton therapy, is a machine which delivers protons with fixed energy. In order to adjust the energy to a level suitable for the treatment depth, the emitted proton beam will be filtered in an energy selection system. Whereas, in the synchrotrons, mainly used for carbon ions, the energy of proton beam can be controlled, and no energy degradation system is required. Therefore, proton beams with narrower Bragg peaks are produced by the synchrotron. Compared to the cyclotron, the generated spot sizes are potentially smaller.

7. Biological aspects of PBT

PBT is still considered as sparsely ionizing irradiation, which has a similar biological effect as photons. The biological aspect in radiotherapy is characterized by the relative biological effectiveness (RBE) which is a conceptual constant determined from experimental data. We also define the biological effective dose or relative biological effectiveness (RBE) weighted, which is the product of the physical dose with the relative biological effectiveness (RBE) factor [13]. The biological dose is expressed as Gy RBE. In clinical practice for the proton therapy, to get the biological effective dose, the physical dose of protons must be multiplied with a fixed relative biological effectiveness (RBE) factor of 1.1. The RBE of protons is defined as the dose of a reference radiation divided by the proton dose to achieve the same biological effect. The proton therapy treatments in almost all institutions worldwide are based on a single value of RBE of 1.1. However, there is growing debate over whether this fixed RBE of 1.1 is still appropriate for protons. In this way, preclinical data resulting from frequent physical and biological experiments stated that there is strong indication that the RBE factor of protons may be variable [14]. In this way, considerable efforts have been made by the international scientific community during the last decades to gain a quantitative estimate on the relative biological effectiveness of proton radiation, yet the question remains open and is a matter of controversy. This uncertainty is supported by the significant differences between reported measured RBE values and those predicted by available biological effect models [13, 15]. Moreover, biological experiments have evidenced RBE dependencies on dose level, linear energy transfer (LET), and tissue type.

In a similar way, it was reported that the value of 1.1 for relative biological effectiveness entails an uncertainty in the determination of the biological dose which is largest at most distal part of the proton track [16, 17]. In two lung cancer cell lines, H460 and H1437, irradiated with protons, the experimental results revealed that the measured RBE profiles strongly depend on the physical characteristics such as dose-mean lineal energy y_d [18]. On the other hand, Harrabi et al. [19] reported that the increased incidence of asymptomatic radiation-induced brain injuries with an increased linear energy transfer (LET) average, observed in this cohort, especially in the distal part of the spread-out Bragg peak, provides strong clinical evidence to support the hypothesis that the relative biological effectiveness of protons is variable and different to the fixed factor of 1.1. Additionally, a thorough RBE review presented average values of 1.1, 1.15, 1.35, and 1.7 at the entrance, center, distal edge, and distal fall-off of the spread-out Bragg peak, respectively [14], indicating the increased RBE toward the distal edge of the treatment field.

In **Figure 8**, the physical dose, the biological dose (RBE-weighted dose), and the linear energy transfer (LET) evolution are represented with respect to penetration depth of proton beam of 220 MeV [20]. This figure summarizes all the results cited

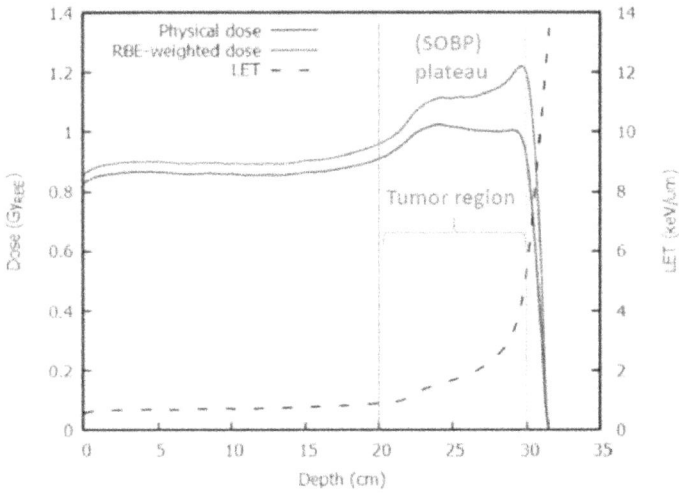

Figure 8.
Physical dose, biological dose (RBE- weighted dose), and the linear energy transfer (LET) evolution versus penetration depth of proton beam of 220 MeV.

above. Firstly, we can identify the tumor area extended from a depth of 20–30 cm, which is also the region of spread-out Bragg peak [SOBP] plateau. The RBE, which represents the ratio (biological dose / the physical dose), remains constant at the entrance, center, and distal edge of the Bragg curve, whereas, it increases in the tumor region [14]. Furthermore, as reported above [19], the RBE increases with increasing linear energy transfer (LET). These interpretations are well schematized in **Figure 9**.

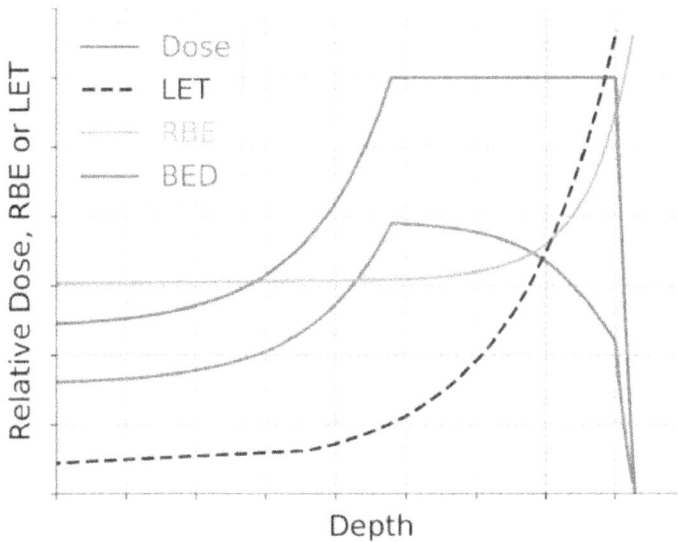

Figure 9.
Schematic diagram of designed dose profile (blue), linear energy transfer (LET; black), relative biological effectiveness (RBE; orange), and biological effective dose (BED; red) with depth [20].

Further investigations will be required to evaluate the quantitative effects of RBE variation on treatment planning and tumor control and toxicity to normal tissues. A better understanding of RBE variability would enable the development of safer and more effective proton treatments.

8. Clinical evidence

Due to its physical and biological characteristics, the PBT can be used in several treatment of the tumor in several parts and organs in the body. Previous studies [13, 14] suggested that patients with head and neck cancer may benefit from PBT. For patients with chest tumors, PBT may be an effective and safe treatment option. In comparison to photons, PBT plans may deliver lower doses to the adjacent organs at risk, such as the esophagus, lungs, and bone marrow, thus improving the therapeutic ratio [21]. In addition, it has been demonstrated that PBT is a safe and effective method for patients with abdominal and pelvic tumors especially localized prostate cancer [16, 17]. Moreover, among the options offered by radiotherapy, PBT is relevant choice to reduce unnecessary irradiation dose in pediatric patients. For this reason, PBT may be useful for the treatment of pediatric cancer [22]. PBT has also a potential benefit in reducing the irradiated dose to normal brain tissue to prevent cognitive dysfunction. Additionally, dose escalation might be possible in radioresistant brain tumors such as high-grade gliomas. PBT may allow dose intensification of chemotherapy by improved hematological tolerance in gastrointestinal, thoracic, and other types of cancer [23].

9. Future advancement of proton therapy

Proton therapy has evolved, and future predictions include smaller systems, more sophisticated proton dosimetry, and devices that manipulate the proton beam. The main challenges of proton therapy are continued miniaturization of proton therapy technology, improved precision of beam delivery, enhanced proton dosimetry computation, and further shaping of the proton beam.

10. Conclusion

Proton beam therapy is the latest kind of radiation therapy, which exerts satisfactory curative effect. In recent years, an increasing number of patients have been treated with PBT worldwide. PBT can achieve a dose distribution that is generally superior to conventional external photon beam radiation. Compared to conventional radiotherapy, PBT proton therapy presents several benefits: Lower risk of radiation damage to tissues, higher radiation dose to the tumor, better likelihood that all tumor cells are destroyed. However, future studies must integrate, evaluate, and manage information associated with PBT, in order to provide patients with the optimal treatment while reducing injury to normal tissues and treatment costs, and to clearly determine which patients may benefit the most from PBT. The relative biological effect of PBT requires further investigation.

Author details

Rafik Hazem[1,2]

1 Laboratory of Coating, Materials and Environment, Umbb, Algeria

2 University M'Hamed Bougara Boumerdes, Boumerdes, Algeria

*Address all correspondence to: wail.rafik@gmail.com

IntechOpen

References

[1] Gaito S, Aznar MC, Burnet NG, Crellin A, France A, Indelicato D, et al. Assessing Equity of Access to Proton Beam Therapy: A Literature Review. Clinical Oncology. 2023;**35**:e528ee536. DOI: 10.1016/j.clon.2023.05.014

[2] Bloch F. Zur bremsung rasch bewegter teilchen beim durchgang durch materie. Annalen der Physik. 1933;**408** (3):285-320. DOI: 10.1002/andp. 19334080303

[3] Bortfeld T. An analytical approximation of the bragg curve for therapeutic proton beams. Medical Physics. 1997;**24**(12):2024-2033. DOI: 10.1118/1.598116

[4] Wilson RR. Radiological use of fast protons. Radiology. 1946;**47**:487-491. DOI: 10.1148/47.5.487

[5] Paganetti H, Niemierko A, Ancukiewicz M, Gerweck LE, Goitein M, Loeffler JS, et al. Relative biological effectiveness (RBE) values for proton beam therapy. International Journal of Radiation Oncology, Biology, Physics. 2002;**53**:407-421. DOI: 10.1016/s0360-3016(02)02754-2

[6] Wilkens JJ, Oelfke U. Direct comparison of biologically optimized spread-out Bragg peaks for protons and carbon ions. International Journal of Radiation Oncology, Biology, Physics. 2008;**70**(1):262-266. DOI: 10.1016/j. ijrobp.2007.08.029

[7] Jette D, Chen W. Creating a spread-out Bragg peak in proton beams. Physics in Medicine and Biology. 2011;**56**(11):N131-N138. DOI: 10.1088/0031-9155/56/11/N01

[8] Rezaee L. Design of spread-out Bragg peaks in hadron therapy with oxygen ions. Report Practical Oncology Radiotherapy. 2018;**23**(5):433-441. DOI: 10.1016/j. rpor.2018.08.004

[9] Schardt D, Elsässer T, Schulz-Ertner D. Heavy-ion tumor therapy: Physical and radiobiological benefits. Reviews of Modern Physics. 2010;**82**:383-425. DOI: 10.1103/RevModPhys.82.383

[10] Farr JB, Moyers MF, Allgower CE, Bues M, Hsi W-C, Jin H, et al. Clinical commissioning of intensity-modulated proton therapy systems: Report of AAPM Task Group 185. Medical Physics. 2021;**48**:e1-e30. DOI: 10.1002/mp.14546

[11] Moyers MF, et al. Physical Uncertainties in the Planning and Delivery of Light Ion Beam Treatments (Report of the AAPM Task Group 2020). Alexandria, VA: American Association of Physicists in Medicine AAPM; 2020. DOI: 10.37206/200

[12] Hagan WK, Colborn BL, Armstrong TW, Allen M. Radiation shielding calculations for a 70- to 250-MeV proton therapy facility. Nuclear Science Engineering. 1988;**98**:272-278. DOI: 10.13182/NSE88-A22328

[13] Mohan R, Grosshans D. Proton therapy – Present and future. Advanced Drug Delivery Reviews. 2017; **109**:26-44. DOI: 10.1016/j.addr.2016. 11.006

[14] Paganetti H. Relative biological effectiveness (RBE) values for proton beam therapy. Variations as a function of biological endpoint, dose, and linear energy transfer. Physics in Medicine and Biology. 2014;**59**:R419-R472. DOI: 10.1088/0031-9155/59/22/R419

[15] Polster L, Schuemann J, Rinaldi I, Burigo L, McNamara AL, Stewart RD, et al. Extension of TOPAS for the simulation of proton radiation effects considering molecular and cellular

endpoints. Physics in Medicine and Biology. 2015;**60**:5053. DOI: 10.1088/0031-9155/60/13/5053

[16] Lühr A, von Neubeck C, Pawelke J, Seidlitz A, Peitzsch C, Bentzen SM, et al. Radiobiology of proton therapy: Results of an international expert workshop. Radiotherapy and Oncology. 2018;**128**:56-67. DOI: 10.1016/j.radonc.2018.05.018

[17] Sørensen BS, Pawelke J, Bauer J, Burnet NG, Dasu A, Høyer M, et al. Does the uncertainty in relative biological effectiveness affect patient treatment in proton therapy? Radiotherapy and Oncology. 2021:**163**:177-184. DOI: 10.1016/j.radonc.2021.08.016

[18] Bronk L, Guan F, Patel D, Ma D, Kroger B, Wang X, et al. Mapping the relative biological effectiveness of proton, helium and carbon ions with high-throughput techniques. Cancers (Basel). 2020;**12**(12):3658. DOI: 10.3390/cancers12123658

[19] Harrabi SB, von Nettelbladt B, Gudden C, Adeberg S, Seidensaal K, Bauer J, et al. Radiation induced contrast enhancement after proton beam therapy in patients with low grade glioma – How safe are protons? Radiotherapy and Oncology. 2022;**167**:211-218. DOI: 10.1016/j.radonc.2021.12.035

[20] Jones B, McMahon SJ, Prise KM. The radiobiology of proton therapy: Challenges and opportunities around relative biological effectiveness. Clinical Oncology. 2018:1-8. DOI: 10.1016/j.clon.2018.01.010

[21] Berman AT, James SS, Rengan R. Proton beam therapy for non-small cell lung cancer: Current clinical evidence and future directions. Cancers (Basel). 2015;7:1178-1190. DOI: 10.3390/cancers7030831

[22] Ahmed KA, Demetriou SK, McDonald M, Johnstone PA. Clinical benefits of proton beam therapy for tumors of the skull base. Cancer Control. 2016;**23**:213-219. DOI: 10.21037/cco.2016.07.05

[23] Sejpal S, Komaki R, Tsao A, Chang JY, Liao Z, Wei X, et al. Early findings on toxicity of proton beam therapy with concurrent chemotherapy for non-small cell lung cancer. Cancer. 2011;**117**:3004-3013. DOI: 10.1002/cncr.25848

www.ingramcontent.com/pod-product-compliance
Lightning Source LLC
Chambersburg PA
CBHW081241190326
41458CB00016B/5865